ON MY MIND

MIND

Editorial Opinions
2008-2010
(Second Edition Revised and Expanded)

By
Roger Hite

July, 2012

Also by Roger Hite

Roger's Run (2012)
Daily Snapshots (2012)*
Decorating the Season with Love (2012)
Dog-Mom (2011)*
The Nun of Camelot (2011)*
Oregon Love (2011)*
From Groundhog Day to Camelot (2010)*
I Still Buy Green Bananas (2010*
The Return to Marlboro (2010)*
Unwrapping Christmas (2009)*
Last Stop before Paradise (2009*)
The Marlboro Incident (2009)*
Buster's View (2009)*
The Loser (2008)*
Buster's Spirit (2008)*
The Iron Butterfly (2008)*
Nesting Among Ducks (2008)*
Cottage by the Sea (2007)*
The Foul Game (2007)
The Five Dollar Fortune (2006)
Vivid Imagination (2005)
The Sister Deal (2004)
The God Switch (2004)
Soul Merchants (2004)
Buster's View (2002)
Mirror Man (2001)
Buster Back at the Wall (2001)
The Twelve Candle Miracle (1999)
What's the Good Word? (1999)
The Ebony Snowflake (1999)
The Art of Awe (1998)
Our Gift (1998)
Buster at My Side (1997)
Buster at the Gate (1995)
Buster at the Wall (1994)

*Still Available In Print

Dedication

To Debby, my wife and best friend!

Preface

My wife Debby and I moved to Eugene, Oregon at the end of January in 2008. For the previous three decades we both pursued careers as hospital staff—Debby was an occupational therapist by training. When she retired she was managing the hospital's Occupational Health Program and several other out-patient departmental functions.

I started my professional career as a university professor, but in 1974 switched careers and moved into the field of hospital administration. Over the years I served in a variety of progressively more responsible administrative experiences, including Director of Organizational and Staff Development, Director of Planning, Assistant Administrator, Corporate Director of Business Development, Executive Vice President, COO. In 2005 we both retired from hospital administration. Debby used her time to pursue her love of birding and gardening. I focused on what had been a parallel passion of mine—writing.

In 1994 I wrote my first small book, **Buster at the Wall: A Golden Retriever Looks at Life, Love, and Death.** The book's success only whetted my appetite to do what I truly enjoyed—putting down in writing my thoughts about a variety of things that were on my mind. The book allowed me to discover a writing voice in the form of our old Golden Retriever, Buster. Each evening he and I would walk about a half mile from our home down the hill to the tiny beach at a place called Rio Del Mar. There Buster and I would sit on the seawall and watch as the surf crashed onto the beach and crawled toward the sea wall. I imagined a dialogue between the dog and myself. It enabled me to put down on paper a lot of what I had on my mind about life and the philosophy I had developed across my lifetime.

The collection of essays taught me how I could share through essay form my opinions and views. It was natural to take such a writing skill and refine it into the discipline required to create editorial opinions for a newspaper format.

In my role as COO for the hospital, I was frequently called upon to ghost write articles on health care topics for the local Santa Cruz newspaper—but ordinarily the material was written for someone else and did not bear my by-line.

It wasn't until 2008 when we relocated from our home on the Monterey Bay in Santa Cruz, California back to the Willamette Valley that I found opportunity to gain my own voice and speak for myself on topics that were on my mind.

Shortly after we arrived in Eugene I found myself compelled to write letters to the editor of the local **Register-Guard** newspaper expressing my opinion on a variety of topics. It was refreshing to no longer worry about being "politically correct" or concerned about reflecting favorably on the organization I led.

In retirement I was free to speak my own mind. But it remained unclear whether anyone thought my opinion was worth sharing with a community at large.
My health care administrative background made me especially opinionated on the controversy surrounding the public perception of the expense associated with the opening of a new hospital. Eugene was abuzz with

conflicting opinions on whether Peace Health had been too extravagant in spending over $500 million dollars to create a state of the art hospital.

I felt so strongly about the subject I decided that instead of writing a short letter to the editor, I would compose a lengthy piece and submit it to Mr. Jack Wilson, Editor of the Editorial Page.

I was pleasantly surprised when he accepted the article and it was published. That was the beginning of my journey into journalism as a citizen of Eugene, Oregon. Over the next three years I published several other articles, many on the topic of health care reform, but a few on topics that were of a more broad interest.

What I have grown accustomed to doing is to spend the time writing an essay that conforms to the newspaper's guidelines of not more than 800 to 900 words maximum. I submit the article and suggest to Mr. Wilson the piece is in my opinion suitable for sharing with the newspaper's readership.

As you will see from the selections in this book, there are at least as many unpublished as there are published opinion pieces! In retrospect, I respect the editorial judgment of Mr. Wilson and am not offended if he elects not to share my opinion with the broader community.

I am pleased however, when I receive an e-mail indicating my opinion will be published! I feel especially blessed to live in a community where I have access to the local newspaper. I am especially proud of my connection with the **Register-Guard** newspaper. Its editorial page is most balanced in the sense it contains both liberal and conservative political views—even though the community of Eugene enjoys a generally politically liberal climate one would expect in a university town!

I decided to collect my essays into a single volume so I can clean out the folders of old newsprint. I can also enjoy putting into print the editorial opinion pieces that did not make it into newsprint. I still think they are worth sharing with family and friends and anybody interested in know what I think about a wide variety of topic.

October, 2011.

* * * * * * * *

(**Author's Notes**: This Second Edition is revised and expanded to contains several more articles on health care that were published in the nine-months between October, 2011 and June, 2012. And, as was the case in the prior edition, I have included a handful of other opinions I felt worth preserving, even though Mr. Jackman Wilson, Editor of the Editorial Page, had reasons for passing over my opinions.

It is appropriate to acknowledge the excellent job Mr. Wilson does when he edits and published one of my submitted guest opinions. He never fails to add or delete words that improve the clarity of my work. It is a skill that otherwise goes undetected by the readership of his editorial page. I am grateful for his professionalism.)

July, 2012

1

"The Local Hospital Controversy"

(**NOTE:** The **Commentary** section of the Sunday **Register-Guard** published this essay on September 7, 2008. The reason I wrote the essay was to express my opinion regarding public concern about spending a huge sum of money on building a new hospital.

I had recently retired from a hospital in Santa Cruz where we were almost begging the corporate office to invest a substantial sum in rebuilding and remodeling an aging facility. It seemed so ironic that when we arrived in Eugene people were being critical of Peace Health for spending what many felt amounted to too much on a state-of-the art facility designed to meet the 100 year need of the Eugene/Springfield community. The article helped me establish my credential as an able writer and a knowledgeable authority on hospital and health care reform topics.)

* * * * * * *

"Hospitals not to blame for rising health care costs"
For-profit and not-for-profit organizations must run a business within a dysfunctional health care market-place.

The competition between Peace-Health and its rival, the for-profit McKenzie-Willamette Hospital, is the same kind of dysfunctional competition I experienced in Santa Cruz, Calif., where I was a health care executive of Dominican Hospital for 30 years.

Like Sacred Heart Medical Center, Dominican is a part of a multiple-hospital system—Catholic HealthCare West—the third largest system in the United States. The for-profit competition in Santa Cruz was--and still is—Community Health Systems, parent company of McKenzie-Willamette. Another not-for-profit competitor in the Santa Cruz market is Sutter Hospitals, a major system that owns many not-for-profit hospitals in northern California.

The distinction between a not-for-profit and for-profit hospital was and still is a semantic blur. All hospitals must make a profit. The distinction lies in what is done with the profit.

All competitors in the health care marketplace want to minimize their investments and maximize their excess revenues over expenses. The for-profit companies pay taxes and are not obligated to provide any community benefit—such as providing elective health care to uninsured patients. Not-for-profit hospitals have a community benefit obligation. They also must reinvest their profits in facilities and equipment instead of paying dividends to stockholders.

In an August 11 letter to the **Register-Guard's** Mailbag, I praised Peace Health for its decision to reinvest $500 million in a local facility instead of vectoring revenues out of the community into more profitable investments in growth markets.

When I speak of "competition," it is important to realize what hospitals are competing over. Health care organizations are not competing for nonpaying patients or state-sponsored Medicaid patients. They are competing for the 10 percent to 25 percent who are private-pay patients. And, in the Medicare population, they are competing for the better reimbursement that the federal government pays for certain categories of medical services such as those provided to orthopedic and cardiovascular patients.

In recent years, as not-for-profit hospitals emulate more of the business tactics and strategies of for-profit hospitals, some government regulators are asking whether society is getting its money's worth by giving tax-exempt status to not-for-profit hospitals. In California, not-for-profit hospitals have an obligation to demonstrate annually the financial benefit to the public provided in exchange for tax-exempt status.

I'm sure Peace Health can easily demonstrate that it provides benefits to the community greater than the equivalent tax bill it would pay if it were a for-profit business. This is due in part to the accounting convention that allows a hospital to claim as a community contribution the expenses associated with its charitable care and the no-pay patients who arrive at the emergency room in need of treatment and hospitalization.

A hospital can also claim a community benefit in terms of the shortfall between what it costs to provide health care to government-sponsored patients, and what the government pays to reimburse hospitals for those services. For many hospitals that have seen the cost of labor and equipment skyrocket while the government cuts reimbursement, this community benefits account-

10

ing number is often huge. The shortfall is made up by shifting expenses to privately insured patients in the form of higher charges.

Get the picture? The more private-pay patients, the greater the cushion against a financial shortfall.

Anyone who has received a bill from a hospital and looks at the difference between the "sticker price" and the actual payment can see the effect of cost-shifting. Nobody pays full retail. The government certainly doesn't, and fewer and fewer insurance companies pay anything close to full retail.

What few people realize is that when the federal government doesn't pay its fair share of costs and cuts its reimbursement, it effectively and invisibly manipulates a hospital's fee system. The hospital becomes a vehicle for taxing privately insured patients with additional charges to cover the shortfall of Medicare patients' costs.

Given this financial reality, one has to wonder why anybody would spend $500 million on a new state-of-the-art hospital. A cynic could say, "Because they could qualify for the financing!"

In a sense, Peace Health has taken out a major mortgage. But unlike the fickle housing mortgage market, the market for constructing a hospital isn't getting any cheaper. And there will never be a future glut of hospitals. To the people who gasp at the $500 million price tag of Peace Health's new RiverBend Hospital, I ask, "How much would it cost to build that facility 10 years from now?"

11

If you want a hint, consider this: I saw the replacement costs for a hospital start at $150 million and grow to well over $250 million in less than five years.

Given the inaction of the McKenzie-Willamette facility to date, one has to wonder if its corporate office will ever justify spending full replacement costs on a facility not located in a growth market.

I would argue that anyone who wants to be a future hospital player in whatever our national health system evolves into needs to ante up now and build. Take heed, Community Health Systems: He who hesitates is indeed lost!

But I can understand why some of the for-profit players may be reticent to put up the dollars now. A plausible strategy is to stick with minimal investments in current facilities and equipment and divest after the cash cow dries up. The strategy would be to avoid investments in a marketplace where there is a strong competitor who is ahead and takes your money to a high-growth, less risky marketplace.

If I were a gambler, I'd bet that CHS keeps McKenzie-Willamette at its current site and makes a minimum investment to maximize its cash flow from this hospital into its corporate coffers. I would guess that such prudent behavior is what its investors expect. CHS is not a bad guy in the dysfunctional health care marketplace. It is simply a prudent player.

CHS, based in Tennessee, is a strong health care organization. It historically built a portfolio of hospitals that were primarily single providers in rural or isolated communities. Such a strategy had a two-fold advantage: It required minimum investment in buildings and equipment, and it allowed for maximum return on investment because there is not competition in setting rates for private-pay insured patients.

Since CHS acquired McKenzie-Willamette and other hospitals formerly owned by Triad Hospital Company, I don't know if its major strategy has changed. The part that certainly hasn't changes is who CHS is positioning its facilities to serve: The most profitable patients, those with private insurance.

Whether you are a for-profit or not-for-profit hospital, there is no opportunity to negotiate prices with the federal government, which is the source of payment for 50 percent or more of the typical acute care hospital's business. The Medicare reimbursement system pays all providers the same, regardless of their status.

So, I hope people can see what is driving the completion among our community's hospitals. The system has created the incentives for competition. Unfortunately, nobody is competing for the uninsured, the low-income patient. Both the for-profit and not-for-profit organizations are trying to run a business within the boundaries of a dysfunctional, inefficient, cost-shifting health care policy.

Whether we acknowledge it or not, we have in America a health care marketplace in which half a dozen major stakeholders are working the system and the rules to maximize the return for themselves at the expense of the total system, and ultimately the patients. But don't single out a hospital, the government, a doctor, a nurse, a union, the pharmaceutical companies or the insurance companies. Recognize the enemy is us—the American electorate. We need to elect and hold accountable legislators who can get all the stakeholders to fashion a policy that works. We will know if it is working when there are no people in need of health care who are denied access.

For anyone who wants to look back at a time when things worked better, one only has to go back to the era when community hospitals were free-standing and unattached to corporate giants. Several decades ago, health care was driven by mission and ministry—not corporate decisions about how to maximize profits by reducing overhead and increasing the productivity of already over-worked health care providers.

In my book **"Cottage by the Sea,"** I wrote about the history of a religious-sponsored private hospital from its inception in 1941 until 1988, when it joined with one of the largest not-for-profit health care systems in the United States, Catholic HealthCare West. In the early history of the hospital there was the close alliance among the care givers—physicians, nurses, and other support staff—and the rest of the citizens and business people in the community.

The contrast to today is stark. Where once we had a truly community-sponsored health care facility, today's version is directed from a central corporate headquarters whose goal is to maximize investment opportunities in growth markets and in the highly profitable segments of individual health care markets.

The solution isn't going to be found in attacking Peace Health for its "over-the-top-opulence,"—which one recent letter writer said contributed to the widening of the chasm between the "haves" and the "have nots."

Suppose Peace Health built a more modest hospital. How would such a facility have contributed to narrowing the chasm between the "haves" and the "have nots?" It wouldn't. The problems would still exist, because our national health care policy isn't working.

The problem is not in the high quality of the physical attributes of a single hospital. The problem is that we lack a national health care policy that creates some form of single payer reimbursement that levels the playing field and eliminates cost-shifting.

The sooner we can elect legislators willing to get all the stakeholders together and fashion a workable health care policy, the sooner we will be able to collectively take pride in one of our community's most valuable assets and stop taking pot shots at isolated stakeholders.

2

"Hospital Put On Hold"

(**NOTE:** It didn't surprise me one bit when the controversy and concern again arose in the Eugene/Springfield when the McKenzie-Willamette Hospital decided to abandon its new hospital plan and to seek another site for its hospital replacement project. The **Register-Guard** published my opinion on the matter in the Sunday, February 8, 2009 newspaper.)

* * * * * * * *

"Clock ticking for McKenzie-Willamette"

I read with interest the Feb. 5 **Register-Guard** article reporting that McKenzie-Willamette Medical Center's owners have abandon plans to build a new hospital on another site and to delay further major remodeling of its existing facility.

There is no good time to invest in a new hospital—it takes a minimum of five years from planning to ribbon-cutting, a time span well beyond normal economic market cycles. By deciding not to build now, McKenzie-Willamette's owners are deciding not to be in acute health care business in the Eugene-Springfield area in the future.

Like it or not, it is only a matter of time until McKenzie-Willamette will be divested or transformed into something other than a general acute care hospital. The clock is ticking. I don't believe it will be next year or the year after, but I will not be surprised to see some kind of transformation during the next decade.

Perhaps this situation illustrates clearly the difference between a for-profit hospital and a not-for-profit hospital. One is necessarily too closely linked to current economic issues to be oriented toward the long term. The other can ignore investor-driven short term expectations and focus on a long range future.

We are surely headed, like it or not, for a single facility community. My reasoning is simple. RiverBend was built so that it already has shell space capacity to expand to well over 500 beds—more than enough to absorb the current capacity of McKenzie-Willamette, and sufficient to meet the community's projected acute-care bed needs well into the future.

Fortunately, whether you are a fan or a critic of Peace Health, the reality is that RiverBend is a first-rate—some say extravagant—facility. It was built with today's construction costs, costs that will surely rise in the future. In a decade, the cost of replicating the $500 million-plus facility will probably be closer to $1 billion. The folks at McKenzie-Willamette know that any further delay will price them out of the market.

I don't blame McKenzie-Willamette's owners and administrators for abandoning plans to rebuild on a new site. The existing facility allows the for-profit CHS to generate a positive bottom line and contribute shareholder value. Adding what would surely be in excess of $150 million in construction expenses in today's dollars would negate the hospital's positive contributions to the parent company's bottom line.

I lament the pending loss of two hospitals in competition—but not because of the economic consequences. Having two grocery stores allows customers to shop where the prices are lower. But it doesn't work that way in health care.

Competition between two hospitals does not create the best consumer price for health care—partly because the government buys a hospital's services at a fixed price for Medicare and Medicaid patients, who represent more than half of a hospital's patients. For those private-pay patients who are insured, some price leverage may be gained by the insurance company if it controls a large enough segment of a hospital's business—but any discount garnered by the insurance company is not passed on to the consumer.

The consequences of a loss of competition will not be economic—the risk will be to the quality and scope of services. Competition in health care drives quality, not price. For example, some physicians may argue that having competing hospitals allows them to put pressure on all facilities by admitting patients to the hospital with the most up-to-date equipment, state-of-the-art technology and the best-trained staff. This leverage is absent in a community with a single hospital.

While Peace Health's leaders can congratulate themselves for having a vision that extends beyond the current bump in our national economy, I am not convinced their success will prove to be in our community's best interest. My concern is not that a lack of competition will restrict choice, or that it will drive up the price of health care. What we all should be worried about is that a single facility is vulnerable to becoming complacent.

How will a hospital prioritize its decisions about services, equipment and staff if it doesn't have to consider the possibility that physicians will admit their patients to a competing facility? Will the hospital be motivated to continue to invest in new technology and expanded programs, or will it vector excess revenues into a parent company that will spend the money in other marketplaces it serves where competition exists?

Will the hospital show the same concern for achieving higher quality and better outcomes if there are not competitors striving to provide quality conscious customers better choices?

It is inevitable that the Eugene-Springfield area will become a one-hospital marketplace at some time in the future. The recent decision by McKenzie-Willamette assures us of such an outcome.

My worry is we could end up with a single hospital that operates from the premise that "average is good enough."

I am going to listen very carefully to Peace Health leaders and how they intend to ensure continuous improvement of quality, now and in the future.

3

"The National Debate on Health Care Reform"

(**NOTE:** Everyone has an opinion on health care reform and how to make the American system better so it can afford to include the 40 million folks who can't afford private health care insurance and who do not qualify for current government-sponsored entitlement programs.

Over the course of a year and a half I made several editorial contributions to the debate that Jack Wilson, **Register-Guard** editor felt worth publishing. The following article appeared in the newspaper on Sunday, July 26, 2009)

* * * * * * * *

"QUID PRO QUO: Can We Accept Responsibility to Improve Health?"

In anticipation of universal health care coverage, I would like readers to use their imaginations and fast-forward to one day after much-heralded legislation is passed by Congress and signed into law. Forty-five million people receive a letter from the President of the United States congratulating them on being entitled to a basic health care insurance plan.

Imagine the President saying:

"My fellow Americans, I am pleased to offer you this coverage. It is coming at great expense to our society. It is the right thing for us to do. I am aware it will be an initial challenge for our current system to provide you access to something that is now your entitlement. I ask you to be patient as we roll out the plan. We will do our best to accommodate your individual situation, regardless of where you reside in this country."

Then the President will unveil an unexpected quid pro quo for each government insurance plan enrollee:

"I want each of you new enrollees to realize there is a corresponding responsibility associated with this new federally mandated health care entitlement. Each of you has a one-year period in which to arrange for a visit to a primary care physician. The purpose of this visit will be to formally enroll you in the government sponsored plan. That means you will be asked to provide a health-care history, you will be given a physical examination and you will undergo a series of risk assessment and diagnostic tests so that you can be assigned into one of several risk categories.

"Once you have been assigned a risk category, you will work with the physician to establish an individual health improvement target. It will be your responsibility to work during the second year of your enrollment to participate in a treatment plan aimed at improving your health status.

"There are only two conditions that can cause you to be dropped from this universal health care plan:

1) If you do not see a primary care physician and establish an individual health improvement target during the first year enrollment period; or,

2) If you fail to participate in the second-year follow-up and ongoing health care assessment and improvement plan created through your first visit to your primary care physician."

"These choices are yours. You are free not to participate and accept the no-coverage consequences. Your fellow American taxpayers are making a major long-term investment in your health and well-being. We as a society are saying it is our obligation to provide basic health care coverage to all—but only if you cooperate.

Your responsibility in turn, will be to participate actively in improving your health. Should you elect not to participate, then you will be dropped from enrollment and not entitled to government sponsored insurance."

Now imagine the backlash that such an authoritarian prescription would create. We'd hear many people say: "Just because I don't take care of myself—no exercise, no dietary restraints, obesity and addictions aside—the government has no right to mandate that I become healthy. I have the right to do what I want with my own body. And I have the right to be insured so that when my body breaks down to the point where I need health interventions, I get such care. All the wealthy, insured people have enjoyed such private insurance coverage in the past without any conditions. I think the government plan should be no different."

Could a transformation of our social attitude towards our responsibility to participate in a system aimed at improving the health status of our population be critical to the success of a universal system? Those who don't want to assume any personal responsibility can opt for the incredibly expensive private plans that will be their only alternative—plans that cannot cherry-pick, and will have to accept noncompliant enrollees and price accordingly.

Of course, it must be said that even if new enrollees graciously embrace these conditions of enrollment, we will still be faced with the daunting task of reducing the costs associated with unnecessary tests, treatments and procedures. But that may prove to be easier than changing the behavior of people who want the benefits of government insurance and not the responsibility of improving and maintaining their own health.

Successful universal health insurance will achieve the goal of improving the health status of Americans only with the cooperation of enrollees. Are we ready for such a challenge?

4

"The Public Debate Heats Up"

(**NOTE:** I got quite opinionated in the public health care reform debate. I tended to want a universal single payer option, but was willing to take an incremental approach to bringing such plan forward over time. The following editorial was published as a guest viewpoint in the **Register-Guard** on Thursday, November 12, 2009.

* * * * * * * *

"Let's Hope Health Reform 'Lite' Just the Camel's Nose in the Tent"

Significantly, most recent news stories are now referring to the health care bill that is coalescing in Congress as "insurance reform." Whatever happened to true health care reform?

As a former hospital administrator, I find it interesting that Congress appears to have decided not to reform health care by taking on hospitals, doctors and the pharmaceutical industry, but to demonize the insurance industry. Why? Because the insurance industry is a pure economic enterprise that makes money by playing the actuarial odds. Unlike health care providers, who actually touch and relate interpersonally with patients, communication with the insurance industry is impersonal and strictly a financial transaction. It is easy to demonize such an industry.

Those of us who favor true reform are clearly going to have to be satisfied with something that falls short of President Obama's desire for a single-payer universal health care system. What we are going to get is a "lite" version of reform in the form of a so-called "public option." Some suggest we call it the "competitive option" or "the public insurance option." Some say states should be able to opt out.

I've come to the conclusion that as much as folks downplay the option and say it isn't critical, it is a critical starting point to true reform. It gets the camel's nose under the tent.

It is hard to know what projections to believe about the potential impact of the public option. In his October 29 column Robert Samuelson told us that the Lewin Group estimated that 103 million people—half the number who currently have private insurance—would switch to the public plan. A few days later a news article told us that the Congressional Budget Office estimates that only about 6 million would sign up for the public option by 2019—only 2 percent of the 282 million Americans under the age 65.

So who to believe? I presume the truth lies somewhere in the middle and it still creates a major financial problem for the funding of our current health care system. Here's the problem that has to be addressed: In order to establish a government sponsored public option, Congress will have to mandate that hospitals and physicians be reimbursed at or near current Medicare rates—which hospital providers will tell you is as much a 30 percent lower than the rates paid by private insurance companies. Because of this price mandate strategy, Congress would supposedly be able to sell and insurance product at a price that is less than individuals and employers pay for health insurance.

So, if Samuelson is correct in many of his assumptions and calculations, hospitals would necessarily have to raise fees to those who remain in private insurance— because it is the base onto which hospitals and physicians currently cost-shift the short-fall created by the Medicare and Medicaid programs.

The degree to which the public option is successful in enrolling folks is the degree to which we will further increase the financial pressures on the existing broken system. There is no free lunch. If the public option is successful, it is going to have to pay providers more than current Medicare rates. A universal single-payer system is clearly superior—if it is well run and held accountable.

Why didn't Obama go for the real reform and support a single-payer system from the get-go? Because he is a smart realist. He knows he is going to have to move the country toward such a goal by increments—hence the public option, the camel's nose version of reform. And I suppose that is better than nothing.

Obama realized he could not pull the plug on the private health insurance industry—a for-profit industry that some estimate has a book value of $250 billion to $300 billion in investor owned stock and employs more than 50,000 people.

It doesn't take a genius to see how the "public option" is the camel's nose under the tent. It opens the way for transitioning over time employer sponsored health insurance into the sector of a government run option—ultimately creating a universal health care system.

If this is the way we have to approach reform, I'll hold my own nose and accept it as a start. But I will still have angst that we are putting more people into a broken system where there is massive fraud and abuse, unnecessary medical treatments, frivolous malpractice suits, uncontrolled pharmaceutical costs and more.

As the bill moves forward, time is of the essence. The Democrats want something before the holiday recess and do not want to drag the debate into 2010 and be a foreshadowing of the midterm elections. Republicans, on the other hand, are gleeful that the off-year elections in Virginia and New Jersey somehow signal that folks are getting frustrated with the current administration's efforts to fashion effective legislation and address the problems that were inherited by the administration.

Don't totally disparage the current public option—however it finally is defined in the massive document moving through Congress. Remember, it is just the camel's nose under the tent. Stay tuned for what happens when the full camel is inside the tent!

5

"A High Compliment"

(**NOTE:** I was especially proud of the response I got from a friend when the following article appeared in Friday, January 22, 2010 edition of the **Register-Guard**. My friend is married to the Dean of the University of Oregon Journalism School. She told me that her husband actually read her much of my article aloud at the breakfast table—something he seldom did! I consider that act a great compliment. I think he especially liked the colorful way I played with the Alice In Wonderland imagery!)

* * * * * * * *

"Through the Looking Glass, Start Anew with Reform Effort"

American politics is getting curiouser and curiouser as we venture down what has become an "Alice in Wonderland"—like rabbit hole of health care reform.

Just as the Mad Hatter is seating all the characters gathering at his tea party—a re-emerging political forum— the White Rabbit scurries through and disrupts the whole affair.

In this version of the story, however, the rabbit is actually Brown.

That's as far as I can stretch the metaphor to make my point about what has happened to our nation's much-needed health care reform legislation. Health care reform has mutated into "political reform."

The Brown Rabbit's message is symbolic: Americans want to temper President Obama's approach. They want him to hear their message and redirect Congress so it can fashion an approach more acceptable to both political parties.

The disruption created by the Brown Rabbit's appearance signals what I hope will be only a temporary pause in the story of health care reform. I'm not discouraged, though, because I don't think Congress or the people it represents have lost any commitment to the goal of improving access to affordable health care for all Americans. The Brown Rabbit signals the need to regroup and get it right, even if it takes another six or nine months.

I know very little about Sen.-elect Scott Brown of Massachusetts. I have no reason to believe he is much different from Obama—an intelligent, decent man with family values and a desire to help solve America's current political and economic problems.

What makes me nervous, however, is not the fact Brown's election breaks the Democrats' filibuster-proof control of the Senate, which I believe was going to assure some form of successful, albeit partisan, legislation. I worry that Brown's amazing rise will lead Republicans to believe he is the answer to their prayers:

a new leader who can challenge the liberal politics of the Obama administration.

Listen to him challenge Obama to two-on-two basketball. It is very populist to have Brown draw the battle line when the president makes a derisive comment about Brown's pickup truck.

It is going to be a sad day for American health care reform if Brown's rabbit-like arrival moves Republican congressional attention away from finding a way to get affordable health care for all and toward using the failure of health care reform as the key to defeating Obama in 2012.

I understand the dilemma Congress faces in the aftermath of Brown's victory. Democrats are fearful of acting on any version of the current bill. Republicans are buoyed by the arrival of the Brown rabbit, who has promised to vote against the bill.

In its current form, the bill is too cumbersome, too filled with special interest compromises and too hard for the American people to understand. It is spurious logic for anyone to conclude "some bill is better than no bill."

It makes more sense to allow both parties to save face so they can get back to the drawing board and refocus on what is needed. As chief of the executive branch, Obama owns the responsibility to lead with such a challenge.

Obama must concede that improving health care access and costs for American is not a sprint. It is going to be a marathon of incremental changes.

The president should challenge both parties to select, prioritize and submit agreed-upon improvements in manageable, bite-size chunks. He should temper his rhetoric and avoid use of the grandiose term "reform" and migrate instead toward the concept of "continual improvement."

In short, we need the image of a different fable: Obama must be willing to play the role of the tortoise, not the rabbit, in the race to improve the American health care system. Dump the notion of a single, sweeping comprehensive reform. There is nothing wrong with making a midstream adjustment and beginning anew with a series of smaller bills that address separately the issues of tort reform, fraud and abuse in Medicare and Medicaid, unnecessary medical treatments, pharmacy costs and insurance product costs and availability.

Obama should not take the bait of pickup truck populism. Let the freshman senator from Massachusetts settle into his seat and become part of the solution. Above all, he shouldn't get into any political one-on-one game with this new rising senator. Obama's goal should be to get his Alice-like Congress out of the rabbit-hole and back to the reality of continually improving the American health care system.

6

"The Medicare Chief Appointment"

(**NOTE:** When I was COO of Dominican Hospital in Santa Cruz, I had the opportunity to work with Dr. Donald Berwick, a Harvard trained pediatrician who founded the highly successful Boston-based Institute of Healthcare Improvement. I had occasion to travel to Harvard with my colleague friend Lee Vanderpool and to consult with Berwick on creating a graduate level curriculum on health care quality for Hospital Administrators.

I was obviously pleased when in early April of 2010 President Obama announced he was nominating Dr. Berwick to head the federal department that oversees the Medicare and Medicaid programs.

On Sunday, April 25, 2010 I wrote the following editorial piece introducing the readership of the **Register-Guard** to the idea it was good to select Berwick for such an awesome responsibility.

* * * * * * * * *

"Medicare Nominee Has What It Takes"
Obama's pick will bring change and improvement to the health care system

With all the controversy surrounding the recently enacted health care reform bill, President Obama deserves kudos for announcing on April 20 that Dr. Donald Berwick is his choice to head the $700 million operations of the Center for Medicare and Medicaid Services.

Berwick is not a high-profile figure, so it's especially important for Oregonians to learn about this extraordinary person. I have seen firsthand Berwick's energetic, hands-on leadership style.

He is not a bureaucrat. He is an advocate of change and improvement in how health care is delivered. He has a track record for demonstrating how health care providers can improve quality while reducing cost.

Berwick, a pediatrician, is affiliated with Harvard Medical School and the Harvard School of Public Health. In 1991, his frustration with his wife's less-than-satisfactory experiences in the health care system led him to create the Institute for Healthcare Improvement.

Over the past two decades, his Boston-based IHI has received worldwide acclaim for deploying systematic clinical quality improvement throughout the health care system. Berwick was awarded the British Cross, the highest honor England can bestow on a noncitizen, for his work with the British National Health System.

In working with Berwick's program, I saw a team work to reduce the common ventilator-acquired pneumonia in the intensive care unit of my hospital, Dominican Santa Cruz Hospital. The ICU went from having the national average infection rate of 2 percent, to an astounding stint of almost two years without a single documented occurrence of the most common hospital-acquired infection!

The results remains one of the classic examples of how Berwick's IHI helped health care providers in hospitals across the country develop and share basic techniques to improve quality and reduce costs. I sat in on bi-weekly conference calls with teams from dozens of hospitals, sharing their insights and improvement results.

Our team of caregivers studies and analyzed such things as the ICU bed angles, as well as the techniques of frequently removing and cleaning the tubes used in intubation. Though it seems counter-intuitive at first, the frequent cleaning of the mucous gunk (my layman's nonclinical description) in and on the tubes led to increases, not decreases, in infection rates.

So, caregivers left the tubes in place during the entire time the patient was on the ventilator—and infections disappeared!

Observations of this type led caregivers to develop plausible, testable hypothesis that improved the results of treatment—improvements that came without the time-consuming double-blind studies used effectively elsewhere in the medical field.

It doesn't take a math wizard to calculate the savings achieved by eliminating additional unnecessary days in an intensive care unit due to hospital-acquired infections.

In the IHI's annual conferences, Berwick created a global forum that allowed physicians and caregivers to share their best practices. I am sure local hospitals in Lane County will testify to the respect given to the leadership Berwick has gained through his institute— and through his challenge to hospitals, issued in 2009,to reduce total resource consumption by 10 percent in three years.

Berwick is a champion of evidence-based medical practice that can be used to improve results for patients while eliminating unnecessary testing. If he can instill his passion for improvement in quality and reduction in costs into the administration of Medicare and Medicaid, the nation's health care programs for the elderly and the poor will insist on putting quality first.

When Berwick undergoes the scrutiny of the Senate Finance Committee in his confirmation hearings, he is going to be the target of some disgruntled Republicans. They will try to associate him with the concept of "health care rationing" and the charge that he advocates "death panels."

If the senators do their homework, they should conclude such attach rhetoric is unfounded. Berwick stands for cost-effective improvements of health care outcomes. He also champions the mantra, "nothing about me without me"—meaning that patients have the right to participate in the decisions about their medical options.

Berwick is not universally popular among health care reform advocates because he has supported compensating physicians on the basis of outcomes, rather than simply being paid for the number of procedures performed. He is also an advocate of creating a non-patient-specific medical information database for providers to validate evidence-based best practice medicine.

Berwick is a major critic of how expensive American health care has become, compared with the costs of other industrialized countries—and says we don't get any added value from spending more of our national wealth on health care.

Opponents of the Obama administration's health care reform legislation are raising legitimate issues, and more will arise as our country deploys the massive changes mandated by the 2000-page piece of legislation. I hope Berwick's appointment does not get bogged down in partisan politics.

The President has made an outstanding choice. Soon after Berwick is confirmed, we will begin to see evidence of his outstanding leadership in improving the quality and the cost of our Medicare and Medicaid programs.

7

"Defending Berwick"

(**NOTE:** It was unfortunate that President Obama did not allow the Senate to hold confirming hearings on his appointment of Dr. Donald Berwick to the head of Medicare and Medicaid programs. Instead, he chose to make a recess appointment and avoid any political clash. I was among those who wished otherwise because I thought Berwick was more than capable of defending his record and his credentials.

As the political controversy continued along party lines, it was clear that Berwick was vulnerable to cheap shots. In mid-July of 2010, a guest editorial appeared in the **Register-Guard** in which a well-intending local activist charged Berwick with advocating "death panels."

I was pleased when on August 2, 2010, I was able to come to Berwick's defense in the following article:

* * * * * * * *

"Some Rationing Critical to Cost-Effective Health Care System"

Gayle Atteberry's thoughtful guest editorial in the July 21 **Register-Guard** reflected genuine misgivings about the appointment of Dr. Donald Berwick to head the Center for Medicare and Medicaid, raising important questions about his views on "rationing" and "death panels." These questions could have been clarified in Senate confirmation hearings.

I was surprised—and disappointed—that President Obama circumvented the Senate and made a recess appointment. If there had been hearings, I am confident Berwick would have been clear in explaining and defending his perspective on using evidence-based medicine to make rational decisions about medical care.

Atteberry's column began with a sound bite from Berwick: *"The decision is not whether or not we will ration care; the decision is whether we will ration with our eyes open."*

Atteberry observed that, *"The Brits have learned that the government cannot afford to provide every British citizen with every needed health service. Cost must be contained, so decisions are made through a 'comparative effectiveness' formula. . ."*

In other words, the British created a process that reflects their best effort to use their health care dollars wisely. The rationing process reflects British beliefs and values—not those of the United States.

I agree with Berwick. Whether we like it or not, resources are limited both in England and the United States. The issue is not whether to ration or not to ration (to restrict consumption), but how to create a sound basis upon which to spend health care dollars.

I have no reason to challenge the facts Atteberry provides about drug restrictions in England, nor do I question the comparative cancer survival rates between the United States and England. England's method of rationing produces poorer results when compared with the United States.

Unfortunately, the column was not able to also show the relative per-capita costs of the American program compared with England. Berwick has been an outspoken critic of the wastefulness of the U.S. health care system. He wants to manage the system so greater value can be obtained from the dollars we spend, compared with other countries that spend less per capita and get better results.

While Berwick may have praised the British for how they manage and allocate their scarce health care resources, Berwick recognizes that the U.S. system is significantly different than England's—especially when it comes to the amount of waste and ineffectiveness in the U.S. system.

If rationing is a "dangerous idea," then it is a dangerous idea whose time has come. In fact, rationing always has been buried in the complex rules and regulations governing what the government will approve for Medicare and Medicaid coverage and how much it will pay.
We need to be less concerned about rationing and more concerned about getting value for the care our government purchases through Medicare and Medicaid.

I am among those who are not frightened by the word "rationing." I do not think slippery-slope reasoning is wise, concluding that rationing is the precursor to what alarmists call "death panels."

We need to probe further into Berwick's priorities for improving the U.S. system before we jump to the conclusion that Berwick's favorable comments about the British system foreshadow some ideal health care plan he is poised to spring on America.

As someone who worked with Dr. Berwick, I have yet to hear him articulate what Atteberry knowingly asserts is "Berwick's ideal health care."

I'm willing to give Berwick an opportunity to propose and defend new approaches before I conclude he has some plan that provides—in Atteberry's words—*"fewer options, less care, long waits and, for many, premature death."*

Those of us who have worked with Berwick and know of the energy he has put into systematic improvement of health care outcomes based on evidence-based best practice approaches to care will judge him in terms of how effective he is in doing the following:

- Addressing the access issues that will be greatly magnified as we expand health care eligibility to millions of previously uninsured people.
- Eliminating billions of dollars worth of fraud and abuse in the Medicare program, giving us more health care dollars to spend on necessary care.
- Establishing a national clinical evidence-based data system that allows best practices to be identified and practiced.
- Reducing ineffective and unnecessary testing and patient care.
- Improving the health status of older and low-income people.

Let's keep an eye on Berwick and see if he can be successful in addressing these issues, and in so doing get us taxpayers a better value for the $700 billion we currently spend on Medicare and Medicaid.

I'm glad for the concerns expressed by Atteberry, but I am more optimistic about what Dr. Berwick will be able to accomplish.

8

"Back to the Drawing Board with Health Care Reform"

(**NOTE:** In early January, 2011, the Republican dominated House of Representatives voted to overturn the health care reform bill passed the previous year under questionable strategies and tactics of last minute Congressional maneuvers by the Democratic Senate and signed by President Obama.

On Monday, January 24, 2011 the **Register-Guard** published the following editorial piece in which I was critical of both parties for gaming the health care issue in an effort to gain political leverage.

* * * * * * * * *

"Only Sensible Health Care Strategy Is to Reform the Reform"

No one should be surprised by last Wednesday's overwhelming House vote to overturn the year-old piece of health care legislation dubbed by many in the unmerciful rhetoric of the public forum as "Obamacare."

Make no mistake. The vote wasn't about how to further improve our system of health care delivery. It wasn't about how to improve the quality of patient services. It wasn't about eliminating the billions of dollars of fraud and waste in the current system.

It wasn't about bringing uninsured people into the health care system. It wasn't even about validating the true cost of the current legislation.

It was about political symbolism. It was about throwing down a gauntlet.

The Senate will not support the House vote, and if it did President Obama would use his veto. The House vote was not an indicator of Congress' concern for the health status of the American people. Politicians on both sides of the aisle are simply setting the stage for the 2012 presidential campaigns.

Where does that leave those of us who saw the current legislation as the first solid step toward some form of universal health care coverage? It leaves many of us with a bad taste in our mouth and the temptation to mutter in disgust, "a pox on both their houses."

Those who rely on government health care entitlements, or who depend on government to regulate insurance so people can afford private coverage, are being told that the expansive plan the Obama administration got past Congress in its landmark legislation was a mistake. It was something the people didn't want, and dissatisfaction with the law led to the overwhelming defeat of Democratic candidates in the 2010 midterm elections.

Yet the fact that the American people are split almost evenly in support of or opposition to the current law does not justify either party throwing out the legislation as unworkable. The challenge is to move forward and modify it so it will work as intended.

The partisan political solution is simple: Throw out the baby with the bath water and start anew. But they won't really start anew until after they've use the rhetoric of health care reform to stake out the Democratic and Republican parties' political positions in the upcoming elections.

Which party is going to address the reality of where we are in terms of improving health care? Is improving health care now relegated to a senseless political game that is really about which party will win the presidency in 2012?

I cynically conclude "yes."

It won't matter if someone like Rep. Pete DeFazio of Oregon provides a workable alternative for those who don't want to be told they must purchase health insurance. He wants such folks to be required to give up their entitlement to Medicaid in the event they need health care coverage.

It won't matter if some creative legislator finds a way to help people with prior health conditions obtained or retain health insurance.

It won't matter if insurance companies are mandated to provide coverage for family members until age 26.

It won't make any difference whether the Congressional Budget Office revises cost assumptions and moves the price tag up or down for whatever new policy is proposed by the Democrats.

Sadly, both parties realize health care policy will be the defining issue in the upcoming presidential campaign. The Republicans will use the House's rejection of the health care reform bill as evidence that our government is spending too much on health care.

Where were these folks when war spending heaped huge debt upon the American people? We afford wars, but balk at affording the "Obamacare" version of national health care.

The Democrats will struggle to salvage as much as possible of their landmark legislation. But right now, those who assess political strategies say the Democrats are on the run.

The Republicans believe they can use the health care issue either to cause Obama not to seek a second term or, should he choose to run, force him to defend an unpopular position.

There is some irony in the fact that when President Bill Clinton ran for his second term, he didn't have to defend his health care legislation. It died on the floor of Congress, never to resurface. President Obama's legislation passed—only to become a seeming albatross around the Democratic candidate's neck in the 2012 campaign.

As a retired health care administrator, I viewed the cumbersome health care reform law as a remarkable step in the right direction. In view of what happened on Wednesday, I say "a pox on both their houses."

Having vented my frustrations, I hope I am wrong and that Congress will focus on doing the right thing—

making the necessary modifications and fashioning bi-partisan compromises to assure our health care is not sacrificed for political expediency.

9

"A Flawed Prediction"

(**NOTE:** On Sunday, April 1, 2012, the following article appeared in the Register-Guard under the headline
"Health care goes back to the drawing board." Nobody at the newspaper could appreciate the irony of the
headline selection. It was the title I used in the earlier
edition of ON MY MIND in reference to the previous
guest editorial I wrote for the January 24, 2011 edition
of the Register-Guard! The other irony in performing
this chapter's addition to my collection was the fact that
I made this addition AFTER I knew the outcome of the
Court Decision!)

* * * * * * * * *

Health care goes back to the drawing board

The U.S. Supreme court is apt to rule that Congress
cannot mandate that people buy insurance if we want to
maintain consistency with the principles of our Constitution.

Those of us who saw the administration's so-called
Obamacare approach as a forerunner of a true national
health care policy should be shaking our heads. Sadly
it is going to be back to the drawing board.

A new Congress will have to find a constitutionally viable way to provide millions of American with access

to health care—and to demonstrate that we are a compassionate country capable of doing what all other industrial countries do to take care of their citizens' health.

I can already imagine the presidential campaign now, providing the Democrate with the cry: "See, we told you the Republicans are out of touch with main-stream America's need for health care." Republicans will champion rhetoric that says, "Fortunately, the system works—and we have protection against unconstitutional laws."

When the Supreme Court divives along its political lines—as surely it will in this landmark case—we are still stuck with the prolem of how to best deal with the problem of providing all Americans with health care.

Is there any segment of the electorate that doesn't want to improce access to health care?

If there is, it has to be a small, selfish, miserly segment. I like to believe we all want to move beyond the mess in which we now seem entalgned.

Why not go back to the original premise that as a country we want all citizens to have access to basic health care, irrespective of their ability to pay for it?

In retrospect, the Obama administration—with both House and Senate in control of Democratic majorities—should have been willint to access a tax on all Americans to pay for some form of national health insurance.

Putting the burden on the insurance industry was an inappropriate solution—something the industry appeared willing to do if we made certain provisions, not the least of which was the must-play mandate for most citizens. In exchange for all players, the industry conceded it would not deny coverage to people with prior health conditions.

Indeed, the administration sought to finess the status uo by using the insurance industry as a vehicle to do Congress' dirty work and enable another form of cost shifting. Instead of shifting the cost of the uninsured to the private sector, thecost was shifted directly onto the shoulders of Americans who for whatever reason chose not to be insured. It wasn't a tax—Congress wasn't willing to be upfront about such a reality. Such a strategy is not apt to be declared unconstitutional.

I don'tobject to "taxing" all Americans for a national health care play—but the government has to be able to control all the associated costs.

In effect, we have to be willing to allow the government to control thecosts of labor, the costs of equirment, the cost of drugs, and to take the profit out of health care for those segments of the private sector that currently game the system.

I have concerns about how such control can be passed on to government, especially when we have made health care business into such a major dimension of our economy. But that is going to be the challenge of revisiting national health care coverage.

The term "tax" was not politically correct during the great health care debate. So, instead of making it clear that we were all going to pay the tab, the administration tried to say that eerbody had to be a player inasmuch as they would buy insurance or pay a penalty. If everybody played, everybody paid—so presumably we could afford the price tag. Sadly we did not know the truecost of Obamacare.

Regardless of the Supreme Court's decision, the estimate of the entire plan's cost was grossly underestimated: In its current form, the Obamacare plan will cost more than $1 trillion. The incredible added financial burden is the new reality Congress must face.

So, as we approach the constitutional showdown over the legality of the administration's attempt to achieve a goal that both political parties have striven for unsuccessfully for at least a generation, it is time to step back and ask: "IF the current approach is unconstitutional, then how do we bring both political parties together after this election and hold Congress responsible for finally providing better access to health care?"

This is really a test of Congress' ability to regroup and find a way to accomplish what the majority of Americans what—a viable, affordable, constitutionally sound and simple approach to health care access for all.

10

"The Supreme Court's Decision"

(**NOTE:** I was among those surprised at the strange twist Chief Justice Roberts brought to the resolution of the case regarding the constitutionality of the ACA. He did as predicted and overruled the use of the Commerce Clause to require all to purchase a minimum health care insurance policy. However, unexpectedly, he allowed the law to remain in tact with the justification it was allowable under the Constitution's authority granted to the government to "tax and spend for the general welfare of all Americans." He also fashioned an interpretation that allowed States to determine if they wanted to accept Medicaid funds to expand their current level of coverage for health care services to the poor in their respective States.

On Sunday, June 24, 2012—the weekend before the Court's ruling—the Register-Guard published my prediction under the headline, *"Examine Reasons behind health care ruling."* Here is the text of that guest editorial opinion:

* * * * * * * * *

"Examine Reasons Behind Health Care Ruling"

If the Supreme Court is true to its past patterns, it will hand down its landmark decision regarding the constitutionality of the Affordable Care Act on Monday.

Not to belabor health care metaphors, but the great question appears to be whether declaring the individual mandate unconstitutional is tantamount to removing the act's life support system, or whether it can survive without that form of financial funding.

A recent poll by The New York Times shows most Americans want the court to overturn the ACA—at least the individual mandate requiring that everybody purchase health care insurance by 2014. According to the Times' poll, only about one in four Americans want the law upheld. Such knowledge, fortunately, is supposedly irrelevant to the court's decision.

The court should not be swayed by whether the public sees the law as good or bd. If the court rules 5-4 to overturn all or a portion of the law, it would not be the first time in history a one-vote margin was a product of justices appointed by one political party (Republican) prevailing over a minority of four justices supporting a law created by the same political party that nominated them to the Supreme Court.

Regardless of the outcome, it will be important for the court to demonstrate that the decision is justified as a result of reasoned analysis and debate—and that as John Adams proudly proclaimed, "We are protected by a government of laws and not men."

I am anxiously awaiting the court's decision, not so much to understand the implications it has for the future of health care in America, but to see whether the justices relied upon arguments and reasoning presented during three days of oral arguments to shape their opinions, rather than issuing a ruling that simply reflects political bias.

I believe the individual mandate will be declared unconstitutional. I believe, though, that the court will somehow dodge the issue of "severability"—that is, the issue of whether an unconstitutional provision in the act invalidates the law in its entirety—and hand back to Congress the challenge of finding a way to preserve some of the laudable aspects of the ACA—what Justice Elena Kagan termed "half a loaf."

If the Supreme Court rules against the current law, it means that it cannot be enforced, but will remain on the books until Congress votes to repeal it and clears the books of what has been rendered a useless law.

This is an important point to keep in mind as the presidential campaign heats up. It elevates the issue of health care reform—perhaps giving it a status equivalent to public concern about jobs and the economy. Both President Obama and former Governor Mitt Romney are going to have to articulate a new vision for what kind of health care people really want—and whoever wins the election in November will have a mandate to take to a divided Congress.

Much has happened since March 23, 2012, when President Obama signed into law the Affordable Health Care Act. States such as Oregon have spent considerable time and resources designing structures to deploy Medicaid reforms. The health insurance industry has dealt with such issues as pre-existing conditions, allowing dependents up to age 26 to remain covered by their parents' health insurance, and banning lifetime maximum insurance limits.

It is not popular to advocate a tax-based assessment on all Americans to fund a replacement for the ACA. But Justice Ruth Bader Ginsburg's idea of funding the ACA in the same way we fund Social Security—by requiring all to pay a tax—is a viable alternative to using the private sector's insurance mechanism as the de facto "taxing" vehicle for funding the program. Hopefully the court's decision will infuse such thinking into the rhetoric of at least one of our presidential candidates and of the Congress the victor will inherit.

The best thing the court can do if it overturns the current health care legislation is to render a decision that somehow transcends the predicted 5-4 split—a decision based on logic and reasoning that preserves the court's role as the protector of constitutional values, and refutes the charge that the justices have become an extension of legislative politics.

11

"Non-Health Care Opinions"

(**NOTE:** Although many in Eugene have come to associate my name in relationship to health care topics, from time to time I have submitted editorial opinion pieces on other topics. One of the first that was accepted was this piece published shortly after I read the obituary of one of my old professors at the University of Oregon.

The obituary said there were no plans for a service—which struck me as sad. I wanted to say something to someone about his influence in my life. I wrote the following essay and asked Jack Wilson if he could connect me with someone who could help me print it in the local newspaper. I was more than willing to pay for the space.

I was delighted when I learned that Jack Wilson knew Bing" and was aware of his passing. He graciously printed my essay on the editorial page.

I was also touched that the morning it appeared in the **Register-Guard** I received a phone call from Dr. Bingham's lifelong friend and companion who thanked me profusely for my kind words.

* * * * * * * * *

"Students didn't skip out of lectures by Professor Bingham"

The July 5, 2009 Sunday Morning **Register-Guard** newspaper contained a small obituary announcing the July 2, 2009 passing of Edwin Bingham at age 89. It was an appropriate time of year for such an event to have taken place for a person who spent his academic professional life immersed in American History.

The thumbnail photo jarred my memory back to the summer of 1971 when Professor Bingham served on my dissertation committee. That was the last time I saw him in person. It was in the hallway of Villard Hall. He and six other faculty members shook my hand and called me "Dr." for the first time after approving my dissertation.

Professor Bingham was for me the commensurate University Professor. He always came to lectures with well-prepared, thoughtful materials organized so they could bring to life some theme or thesis he had teased from his studies of American History. Even though I took his trilogy of courses during my third-year of graduate studies, I repeated two of the courses the following year and found they were once again freshly researched and expanded. He was definitely not using "dog-eared" lecture notes. He had a passion to continually improve his materials and presentations. He constantly experimented with multi-media ways to enliven presentations long before personal computers and electronic technology currently available to modern faculty.

He was one of those professors hard to fit into an academic slot—he resided in the History Department—but he transcended the label of history professor because he wanted his story to get beyond the common perspectives of economic, social, or political history. Professor Bingham relished looking at the American experience as a many-faceted diamond. He wanted students to see how art, music, literature, drama, architecture, poetry, religion, industrial inventions, all created the awesome American experience. He called his popular three-quarter sequence of classes "American Intellectual History."

Although most memories of my time as a graduate student have faded, I still recall vividly the assigned reading and preparation I completed so I could fully enjoy a lecture by Professor Bingham. He introduced me to Samuel Eliot Morrison and the foundation of the puritan traditions—but through an understanding of the early poetry, the religious themes, the crafts, the architecture and the paintings of the time—not just chronology of significant events and dates—but the passion that drove such events. His course was one of the most popular in the history department. He filled a large lecture hall with undergraduates as well as graduate students.

Years after my Oregon experience when annual business responsibilities took me to Washington DC, my recollections of Bingham's outstanding lectures resurfaced. The moment I stepped into the Smithsonian Museum of Natural History I realized what a great gift I'd received from Professor Bingham. In a classroom in Eugene—about as far away from the Smithsonian as one could get and still be in the United States—he brought to me a rich understanding of our American cultural traditions—I wondered how much greater it might have been had he been able to walk us through the museum and use its awesome displays to illustrate the themes he found in his scholarly journey into American Intellectual History?

He would have been a great curator of that awesome display! As I walked through the Smithsonian I found myself recalling things Professor Bingham taught me years earlier.

Professor Bingham had a soft-spoken, almost shy demeanor in his lecture style. There was a humility in the thoughtful way he teased from art, music, poetry, architecture, etc. the story of our American experience and organized it into thought provoking lectures.

I still recall how he brought to life the intellectual concept of "healthy provincialism" and how such a theme was such a vial component of the American experience. He used a Sinclair Lewis character from BABBIT to illustrate how vital small-town "booster-ism" was in the American intellectual experience.

I might have been inclined—from time to time—to skip some classroom lectures to bone-up for an exam in some other subject area where I was being challenged—but I never missed a Bingham lecture—not in the five quarters where I enjoyed his presentations. They were too good to miss.

A year-and-a-half-ago my wife and I returned to Eugene after a thirty-year hiatus. On several occasions I've meandered around campus and reminisced about my years as a graduate student.
I recently asked a retired history professor I met at a meeting, "What ever happened to Professor Bingham? Is he still alive?" His reply was "Yes. He's still with us. I'm sure he'd enjoy a visit from a former student."

Sadly, I didn't make that visit. But this morning when I read the obituary I realized time had woven him into my personal history. I will continue to appreciate the significant contributions Professor Bingham made to my life. Thank you, Professor Bingham.

12

"In Praise of Philanthropy"

(NOTE: Shortly after we relocated in Eugene, I was asked to join the Board of Directors of Catholic Community Services of Lane County. Given my background in healthcare and my long time affiliation with a Catholic not-for-profit health care ministry, I welcomed the opportunity to serve on that local agency's board.

On December 6, 2009 I wrote a guest editorial praising the work of the agency and encouraging community folks to support the agency's mission and ministry as it moved into a new distribution center building.)

* * * * * * * * *

"Catholic Group's Ministry Expands, Offering Services to All"

The 19th century Baptist minister Russell Conwell was best remembered for two things: founder of Temple University in Philadelphia, PA, and his inspirational lecture ACRES OF DIAMONDS.

His lecture was first published in 1890. The theme was simple and was introduced by Conwell in an anecdote about a man who sold all his property and went off to find diamonds. The new owner of his home discovered that a diamond mine was located right there on the property. The inspirational message resonated with audiences who sought reassurance that through hard work, service, and virtue success was possible without going to exotic far-away places in search of adventure and challenges. Conwell travelled the world giving the lecture more than 6,000 times. "Drop down you buckets where you are; dig in your own back-yard!"

For those who want to make a difference when it comes to the challenge of mitigating world hunger, Conwell's message should resonate. The acres of diamonds metaphor aptly describes the gem that has now been planted on .61 acres of land on 6th street in Eugene. For those who want to make a difference when it comes to feeding the hunger, one can "drop your bucket where you are."

I was raised in the Baptist Christian religious tradition so from an early age I was introduced to the story about Jesus Christ performing the miracle of multiplying the fishes and loaves of bread so they could feel the thousands who had gather to hear Christ preach his sermon. As an adult, I also learned that scholars have offered various other interpretations of what happened that afternoon in Tabgha, near the Sea of Galilee when the masses were fed by Jesus.

Some say the fishes and loaves were actually the generous sharing of all who had come to hear the sermon. It was the contributions of the community of followers who shared what they had with their neighbors. I prefer to believe the former—but I understand how for non-believers the latter description is more aligned with their view of the world.

Hunger in the world—regardless of one's religious views—is a great tragedy. I have always argued the greatest crime of humanity is starvation. There is no scarcity of food in the world. It is a distribution problem. No one in the world should go without food—but when one considers the problem of world hunger it can be overwhelming to an individual who asks what difference can one person make? That's why those who want to make a difference have an opportunity to "drop down their buckets" right here in Eugene.

That is the mission of the Catholic Community Services of Lane County—and has been such for more than fifty years. On December 7th, the agency is occupying a new building on 6th Street. It will serve as one locus for the distribution of the seven tons of food that the community contributes and is distributed to the needy each week through the agency.

While CCSLC does more than distribute food—by helping with rent subsidies, parent counseling, energy subsidies during winter months, and a variety of other social services, central to its operations is the awesome job it performs each week as it distributes food in the same loving spirit of Jesus Christ.

I am a non-Catholic Christian member of the Board of Directors of CCSLC. I was attracted to supporting the ministry because in my mind-eye I likened it to the Christ miracle of multiplying the resources and feeding the masses.

I know there is no miracle involved in this ministry of feeding the hungry in the spirit of Christ. There is, however, a great satisfaction that comes from knowing that I am spending the currency of my life addressing the issue of hunger that exists right here in our Eugene/Springfield community. Through my support of the CCSLC I have "dropped my bucket down where I am." I believe I am making a difference right here at home.

I know these are hard times for many. But somehow people who have some resources appear more than willing to share their scarce resources with others. I was amazed recently as I participated in the fundraising phone-a-thon and listened to people pledge small $5 and $10 dollar pledges. Such generosity enabled CCSLC to raise over $71 thousand dollars thanks to an anonymous matching grant of $30 thousand dollars.

CCSLC took the risk to improve its operations by moving from its current crowded location on 7th street to the new facility on 6th that will open officially on December 7th. I hope many will find time to stop by during the open-house celebration and see all the resources that have been gathered to serve the needs of our community. I hope leaders of all denominations will feel comfortable gathering food throughout the year and donating it so it can be distributed through this effective system created at the CCSLC agency. I hope, too, that all religious leaders in our community will feel welcomed to refer those in their congregations to use the services of this diamond in our community.

13

"Opinion on Civic Duty"

(**NOTE:** I was especially annoyed when I arrived at the courthouse in downtown Eugene to fulfill my responsibility to serve on a jury. It was the first time I'd been summoned for better than two decades. I was stunned that only about a third of those summoned serve actually appeared. That event prompted the following editorial opinion published on Sunday, December 20, 2009.)

* * * * * * * * *

"Be a Soldier: Show Up for Jury Duty"

Recently, over 300 persons were summoned to the Lane County Courthouse to participate in the jury duty selection process. Sadly, only about a third of those summoned appeared.

A young Army Ranger I know will soon ship out of Fort Lewis on his second tour of war duty. His first was in the sweltering heat of Iraq. His second will be the frigid winter months that will be spent in the mountains of Afghanistan. He is unaware of the trial I am about to describe or its relationship to his duty as a soldier.

I hope readers will realize, though, these two seeming isolated events are indeed connected.

I was one of 117 people who did appear for jury duty selection. Throughout the morning I listened and watched. At first, I was among the many prospective jurors holding my breath as the attorneys moved through the selection process—hoping I would somehow avoid the inconvenience of serving.

Several people appeared to contrive answers designed to prejudice themselves as good juror candidates. Smirks appeared on some faces as dismissed candidates exited the courtroom, relieved they had "beaten the system."

Halfway through the jury selection process, one man revealed he had a physician's appointment the following morning. His doctor was going to evaluate him for a heart monitor. When the judge interceded and offered the man release, the man was adamant.

"No, it is not a problem. If selected, I can move my appointment. It is not critical."

That's when I began hoping I would be selected to serve with this older gentleman. He was my hero of the day. It was a lesson in the honor of duty.

When the trial began jurors were introduced to the underbelly of the methamphetamine drug world. The defendant was a bundle of social problems. He was homeless. He was scruffy looking. We learned he had high blood pressure. He was visibly uncomfortable. His face was etched with evidence of alcohol and perhaps drug abuse. If left to judge him on how he appeared and acted, it would have been a unanimous "guilty" decision!

But we had to judge a complex case of circumstantial evidence—an argument that wove a web of seemingly small, unrelated items of evidence into a chain of reasoning leading to a guilty charge.

When the jury received the case, twelve strangers from diverse backgrounds engaged in reasoned dialogue. We did our duty. It was painful because we concluded that irrespective of our personal feelings, the evidence did not meet the tests the judge instructed us to use.

We returned to the courtroom. Our lead juror handed our verdict to the bailiff. We found the defendant not-guilty on the charge of possession and on the charge of intent to sell almost an ounce of meth that was found under the car seat where he was sitting when detained at 4:00 am in the morning in Springfield.

I found it hard to look at the district attorney's face. He had failed in his efforts to remove someone from society he felt was guilty of selling drugs. The DA's role, however, was not to judge guilt or innocence. His role was to present evidence. It was the jury's role to judge the evidence.

On the drive home I struggled to put my feelings in perspective. I realized the district attorney had nothing to be ashamed about. He had done an outstanding job of fulfilling his duty.

I didn't feel good about the trial's outcome. The defendant will rejoin the meth user and dealer underbelly of our community. It was a terribly expensive and time consuming process. It was, however, our collective duty as a society to afford the defendant his day in court.

I finally put it all in perspective when I remembered my Army Ranger friend's upcoming departure. He was fulfilling his duty by once again going to a dangerous place in the world to fight the enemies of our way of life.

Then I discovered what was really bothering me. I was angry at the couple of hundred people who ignored the summons.

When we feel put-out because of our obligation to fulfill a duty of citizenship, we should think of our soldiers. We are blessed with all- volunteer military forces made up of people who have responded to a sense of duty. It is because of our soldiers' fulfilling their sense of duty we are able to maintain a society that allows people –even those living on the margins of society—to have their day in court.

The next time you receive a summons to appear for jury selection think about what I am saying. View your summons as an invitation to honor your duty of citizenship. Contrast the inconvenience you might perceive with the hardships a soldier endures when he or she responds to the call of duty.

Our court system works because people show up. Shame on those two-hundred plus people who didn't appear—or who appeared with concocted excuses not to serve.

14

"More Praise for Philanthropy"

(**NOTE:** I have occasionally been impressed with local activities that serve the good of the community. In my role as a director on a local not-for-profit agency, I am especially interested in encouraging community philanthropy. That was the purpose of this guest editorial.

* * * * * * * * *

"Step Up to the Plate for Charity"

The Random House Webster's College Dictionary defines philanthropy as *"altruistic concern for human beings, especially as manifested by donations of money, property or work to needy persons or to institutions advancing human welfare."* The definition fits what's happening in Lane County.

In the first century, the ecumenical patriarch of Constantinople, St. John Chrysostom, wrote: *"If you have two shirts in your closet, one belongs to you—the other belongs to the person who has no shirt."*

Now, more than ever, we need to celebrate and give thanks for our community's philanthropic spirit.

Sure, things are tough economically. Everybody knows that. But consider what the people in the hard hit restaurant business are doing: donating their time and resources to participate in the upcoming Chefs' Night Out.

Fifty local restaurants, wineries, microbreweries and caterers combine their concerns and participate in the event sponsored by King Estate's winery at the Hult Center on Tuesday. The event enables attendees who may otherwise be cutting back on dining out to purchase tickets and help raise funds for Food for Lane County.

Special appreciation is due the organizers and all the volunteers who donate to such a worthwhile cause. Of course, it is just one of the many examples of our community's philanthropic spirit.

Now is the time to celebrate and recognize how blessed we are to be a part of such a community philanthropy. It is time for each of us to look in our own closets— metaphorically and literally—and generously share in proportion to what we have.

The restaurant business owners and their staffs understand that in hard times philanthropy is needed even more than in good times. Giving a piece of one's resources during a banner year is certainly laudable—and easier than in hard times. Giving when strapped requires optimism about the future and a willingness to help those who are hard hit to survive.

You don't have to be rich to engage in philanthropy; all it requires is a willingness to share in proportion to your own resources and blessings. Some have likened philanthropy to "community tithing"—a secular opportunity for all individuals in our community to set aside a portion of their resources and direct it towards programs such as the Chefs' Night Out fundraising event.

What motivates philanthropy, especially during these times of global economic uncertainties? A generous spirit; an optimistic outlook on life; and a passion to act now!

Now more than ever, we need to express our gratitude for all those philanthropist in our community who keep alive the spirit of giving—the restaurant owners and their employees, and other small businesses and individuals, who give of time and resources. Philanthropy is the spirit that will see us through these uncertain times and help our community rebuild its economy.

We need to be thankful there are people who champion optimism about a brighter future.

We need to be thankful there are people willing to act now!

On a recent Sunday I listened to Ben Cross, the pastor of the First Baptist Church in Eugene, deliver an insightful sermon on the topic of community giving. His thoughts were inspired by the scriptures in the book of Acts, where Paul described the Christian church during the first century of its formation.

The sermon reminded us that all wealth is God's wealth—and God gave us the gifts and talents that enabled us to accumulate wealth and possessions. God also gave us membership in communities—its churches, neighborhoods, and workplaces. With such membership comes the obligation to share resources for the good of the various communities in which we participate. In the final analysis, when we live in community "we are all in this together."

Support Chefs' Night Out and the other worthwhile acts of community philanthropy. The restaurant owners, wineries, microbreweries and caterers and their employees found an extra shirt in the closet. How many shirts remain on hangers in your closets? Let use the opportunity of this economic crisis to unleash the full potential of our community's philanthropic spirit.

If not now, then when?

15

"Standing on Principles"

(**NOTE:** It is probably inevitable that when one joins a not-for-profit service organization board of directors they are apt to confront controversy because people have different ways of looking at the world and how an organization's mission should be served. When I became President of the Board of Directors of Catholic Community Services of Lane County it was a member organization of United Way. It had a long tradition of receiving funding from the agency. However, when another member agency—Planned Parenthood of Southern Oregon—began providing abortions, there was a split of opinion on the CCSLC Board regarding continuing association with United Way.

The following article was published in the **Register-Guard** on Friday, December 31, 2010. It was co-authored with a fellow board person, Ms. Sue Paiement. It was our effort to share with the community the rationale behind the decision to withdraw membership from United Way.

* * * * * * * * * *

"Catholic Agency's Services to Continue without United Way"

Register-Guard reporter Diane Dietz did a solid job on Dec. 28 of reporting the facts surrounding Catholic Community Services of Lane County's decision to withdraw from United Way funding. She did so without input from Catholic Community Services' board president and its spokesman, Roger Hite, who was out of town for the Christmas holiday.

Our purpose here is to share further background and to make clear that Catholic Community Services is not ceasing to offer the services outlined in Dietz's article. Instead, it is working to replace the funds it had received traditionally from United Way until Planned Parenthood modified its program and began providing abortions to Lane County residents.

As a result of a November 22 board decision, Catholic Community Services announced it regretted it had no choice but to end its relationship with United Way of Lane County, effective December 31.

When good community-focused organizations such as Catholic Community Services and United Way sever a long-standing relationship, you can be sure, as radio commentator Paul Harvey used to say, it's worth hearing "the rest of the story."

For many years United Way supported the valuable services provided by Catholic Community Services. It treats clients (Regardless of religious affiliations) with an abundance of respect. It provides needed social services as described in Dietz's article and distributes seven tons of food weekly. It has carried out its mission in the spirit of Jesus Christ for the past 50 years.

United Way provided in excess of $10,000 monthly to support Catholic Community Services' programs. Many earmark their United Way campaign contributions for use by the agency.

We are first and foremost Christians who believe that helping the poor is an ecumenical responsibility transcending religious denominations. As board members, we consider the advice of the Rev. John Vlazny, archbishop of Portland. He had not expressed any concerns until last year, when Planned Parenthood of Southwestern Oregon announced it would begin providing the so-called "medical abortion" pill to its clients.

The archbishop then sent a letter to our board, and it was unequivocal: "The only way that CCSLC could remain in United Way as a Catholic agency would be that no agency which provides abortion also be a part of United Way.

For the archbishop, this issue was déjà vu. Several years ago, the same issue surfaced in Portland. The result was that Catholic Charities of the Archdiocese of Portland withdrew from United Way. The archbishop reasons that he must be consistent and apply the same logic to Lane County's circumstances.

Communications flowed back and forth for several months with the archbishop, United Way, Planned Parenthood, Catholic Community Services and many other concerned parties.

At its November 22 meeting the Catholic Community Services board voted to follow the directive from the archbishop. We informed United Way that the only way Catholic Community Services could participate in

United Way was if United Way established and enforced a specific policy excluding providers of abortions.

United Way membership and funding of agencies is a local matter. There is no national policy, for example, prohibiting abortion providers such as Planned Parenthood from being member agencies. As a frame of reference, fewer than 25 United Way organizations out of more than 1,000 across the country have Planned Parenthood as a member agency—but the choice is local.

As a final effort to find a local solution, Priscilla Gould, executive director of United Way of Lane County, formed a task force at United Way. In earlier discussions, United Way indicated it did not solicit funds for the purpose of providing abortions. It was clear, however, that some in the Catholic Church leadership felt uncomfortable with a Catholic-sponsored organization helping raise funds for abortions via United Way's campaign. In Dietz's article, Bud Bunce, the archbishop's spokesman, provided the historical background behind the archbishop's position.

The executive directors of Catholic Community Services and United Way both deserve kudos for their tireless work to fashion a solution that would meet the needs of Catholic Community Services and could be supported by the diverse views of both organizations' board of directors. Such a solution did not emerge.

The archbishop told our board in his most recent letter: *"It is now my determination that CCSLC must terminate its relationship with United Way of Lane County no later than November 30, 3010. Otherwise, I shall terminate the memorandum of agreement and your status as a Catholic agency on that same date."*

As board members, we side with the poor and vulnerable people who want food, not theology. But we also remain respectful of those who are grounded in theological arguments. Unfortunately, when the issue falls into the pro-life vs. pro-choice religious debate, there is no middle ground for compromise.

We are concerned about how the decision affects the future of our mission. Our budget is tight. Giving up the United Way funds will have at least a short-term impact on our agency.

The board makes no apology for standing up for expressing our beliefs in this matter. Our vote was not unanimous—but it was a strong majority vote.

Neither United Way nor Catholic Community Services are the bad guys in this situation. Sadly, both were ineffective in finding common ground for continuing their relationship.

Now that readers know "the rest of the story," we hope they will help sustain the important mission of Catholic Community Services independent of the funding it received from United Way.

16

"Arguments over Pledge Serve Crucial Objective"

(**Note:** This opinion was published on July 13, 2011. It reflected my strong reaction when I heard about the local controversy in which City Council alleged voted to not say the Pledge of Allegiance before City Council meetings. Actually, the story was distorted as it went almost viral after a story broadcast on Fox News. The truth of the matter was that the city council actually voted to begin saying the pledge at least four times a year to show respect for such national holidays as Memorial Day!)

* * * * * * * *

Many traditions mark our national pride in the Founding Fathers' bold decision to declare our independence from the British empire on July 4, 1776. The Pledge of Allegiance is one such tradition—even though some now question whether it's time to modify the ritual.

The Register-Guard has published several opinions reflecting both sides of the arguments over saying the pledge at Eugene City Council meetings.

Pledging allegiance to the flag is a symbolic act designed to show respect for our country—like removing one's hat and standing while our national anthem is sung at sporting events.

The controversy over the pledge, however, is symptomatic of something more deeply rooted in our political process. My thesis is this: when local government faces monumentally complex issues—such as budgets, unemployment, transportation, homelessness, drugs, crime, education funding and health care access—we should not be surprised when procedural topics such as whether to pledge or not to pledge appear on the agenda.

Such topics, though hotly debated by impassioned and often contentious advocates, lend themselves to easier resolution. They often are based on the advocates' beliefs and values, not on who has argued most effectively on the basis of evidence and reason. The house is divided on the basis of beliefs and values. In a community that prides itself as being "politically correct," debates over process issues often affirm the solidarity of shared values and beliefs.

In the democratic process, there is often a long journey between identifying a problem and deploying a solution. Indeed, our two-party system often polarizes the country over the choice of an appropriate solution. Politics, of course, is supposedly the art of compromise.

The Eugene City Council received negative feedback from some national news media for its decision. If someone asks me whether the council's compromise solution was right, I am reminded of something U.S. District Judge Michael Hogan recently admonished folks in a mediation in which I participated: *"We found an imperfect solution in an imperfect world."*

The flag pledge issue is now behind the City Council. It can now focus its attention solely on the other urgent problems facing Eugene. But do not be too critical of the council for taking time to argue about the appropriateness of the pledge at its meetings.

The debate served a useful purpose. If you are having difficulties in making decisions about policies and outcomes, then you should focus occasionally on an issue of procedure or process. At least you can have the satisfaction of using the democratic process to reach a decision—even if it is not consequential in resolving the real issues we face as a community or a nation.

A while back, I made a choice when the issue of having an American flag and reciting the Pledge of Allegiance surfaced at an organization to which I belonged. I am of a generation that said the pledge each morning in public school. At my local organization meeting, I was amazed at the passion on both sides. These were all fine, responsible, good people. Several members did not want an American flag present at meetings. Some also did not believe we were "one nation, under God, indivisible with liberty and justice for all."

I felt uncomfortable in such an environment. I respected the impassioned advocates of doing away with the flag and the pledge. I left the organization and focused my volunteer work elsewhere in the community.

In a sense, I made a process decision and deployed it! I didn't want to be a part of the organization's meeting process—a decision I made independent of my feelings about the good the organization could accomplish through its programs.

The Eugene City Council debate was not about who is a true patriot or who is loyal to the ideals upon which our country was founded. The debate was over what I call democratic process therapy. It was designed to see how the house was divided on the basis of values and beliefs. You have to draw your own conclusions as to whether you share the same values.

Regardless of which side of the issue people are on, I hope our community can agree that Eugene and the United States of America are placed where we are free to express view on both sides of all issues. Let's all pledge to move beyond process therapy. Let's pledge to fill the local and national political agenda with sustentative topics, and fashion workable compromises between our highly polarized two parties.

On Monday, we celebrated Independence Day—a time to affirm that we are all together in our desire to remain a strong, viable democracy capable of finding solutions to our complex challenges.

17

"Borders Closure Indicator of Change"

(**Note:** I was among those saddened by the announcement that the local Borders book store was closing—but the event did not surprise me. I explained my perception in a guest editorial published in the July 24, 2011 Sunday edition of the **Register-Guard.)**

* * * * * * *

I don't want to say I am stunned by the recent announcement that all Borders book and music stores are closing and the company is quickly liquidating its stock. It follows a trend easily spotted by those of us in the book-writing business, either as a hobby or as a profession. I will miss spending leisurely Saturday mornings grazing through books at the Borders store in the Oakway Mall in Eugene—especially during the holiday seasons, when I search for unique books as gifts for friends and family.

I see a parallel with the transformation that digital technology brought to the movie rental business, as Blockbusters gave way to Netflix. The capacity to transform a book into an electronic file and to print individual copies forever changed the publishing industry.

According to the American Booksellers Association in May 2010, the number of independent booksellers nationally declined to 1,400 from 3,250 in the past decade. Independent stores account for just 10 percent of book sales. Chains such as Barnes & Noble's and Borders clung to 30 percent of the market. Superstores such as Costco, Target and Wal-Mart claimed about 45 percent, though they carry significantly fewer titles.

It is useful for those who lament the passing of Borders to understand some factoids about publishing: The average book in print in the United States sells fewer than 2,000 copies in its lifetime. Forty percent of all books brought from print-on-demand producers are purchased and distributed by their authors.

Most readers do not realize how Lightning Source was founded in 1997—and through its incredible growth, now prints on demand 1.5 million books a month. Lightning is part of Ingram Book Co., the biggest U.S. book wholesaler. Almost all bookstores and libraries in the United States order books from Ingram. Lightning's books are not printed in large lots, but are distributed through smaller print-on-demand orders. POD is now the rule, and not the exception.

Historically, a publishing company's dream was to have 10 authors selling a million books each. Now Bob Young, founder of the POD company Lulu, wants a million authors selling 100 books each!

Though I am saddened at the passing of Borders, as an author who currently has more than a dozen titles selling on Amazon.com I realize I am as much a part of the problem as I am prospering from the new reality. I realize that book publishing as we have known it has changed forever—for better or worse.

What happened? There was a time when large publishers competed to find best-selling authors and promote their work on nationwide book signing tours. Publishers scanned the horizon for writer's whose works could be promoted, seeking profit through the printing and distributing of best-sellers. Wannabe writers sent letters and manuscripts to agents who sorted through the volumes of inquiries in search of the next best-selling book. It was—and still is—a highly competitive market; few writers realize their dream of making a living as an author.

What many don't realize is that most books available in Borders and the other national chain book stores are not printed and stored in massive warehouses and shipped to be stored on bookstore shelves. More and more books are simply being printed on demand.

Print-on-demand technology, combined with Internet distribution channels, has enabled writers to circumvent the traditional publishing bureaucracy and get books to market with virtually no upfront expense for the writer or the electronic copy distributor. That doesn't mean high quality books are not commingled with error-filled, poorly edited and badly formatted books. A certain level of professionalism has vanished with this rush to the POD publication alternative.

I am an independent author who writes from my home. When I complete a manuscript, I upload it to CreateSpace—one of the many reputable book producers. It is simply a book producer, and does not focus on marketing and distribution. CreateSpace leaves that task to companies such as Amazon.com.

Instead, the company helps the author produce high-quality, professional looking books—and it has the ability to print, sell, and make a profit distributing one book at a time. CreateSpace doesn't need a Barnes & Nobles storefront, or a Borders, or a Waldenbooks, with their overhead expense.

Instead of paying a publisher to make a 1,000-copy run of a book and storing the boxes of books in my garage until I can figure out a way to get them into a distribution network, I now order my own author's copies at a discount and make other copies available through the Internet distribution process managed by Amazon.com.

There is incredible efficiency and speed n the whole process. I have no upfront cost of production, and for the cost of a single proof copy delivered to my own doorstep within a week after I complete the upload, I have a book with an International Standard Book Number (better known as ISBN) available nationally and globally to potential customers. My investment" Less than $10, plus shipping of the proof.

Amazon.com has created a profitable venture with print-on-demand businesses. After all, the companies such as CreateSpace can make a profit printing each book they send to the writer to distribute and market. Any book purchased through Amazon.com does not cost Amazon anything to print, store and distribute.

Instead, the customer pays all the production and shipping costs. There is not store overhead, and the book can be delivered directly to the customer's front door in a couple of days.

But I still lament the loss of Borders. I like the high touch of a book store. I look forward to seeing how such a model can be resurrected in our modern economy. I am optimistic somebody will step up and find a way to make a bookstore a viable model in the modern publishing world.

It is with sadness I say goodbye to the Borders of the world!

18

"Old Hospital Is a Burden PeaceHealth Must Shed"

(**NOTE:** The topic of health care was a front page story in which a reporter wrote two excellent stories comparing the financial challenges facing both local hospitals. An additional story about PeaceHealth asking for an extension of its plan to renovate the old Sacred Heart facility now knows as the University District Hospital also accompanied the feature stories.

I initially wrote an editorial that was not published (it appears later in this volume as "Beyond Profitability.") The editorial that appears below was written the evening after I sent the piece on profitability to the **Register-Guard.**

Paul Neville, the associate editor of the editorial page e-mailed me and asked if he could publish the piece that appears below. I suspect he realized it would provoke the kind of response evidenced by the immediate e-mail responses the newspaper received on Thursday, September 8, 2011. The two-dozen responses demonstrated to me that feelings still run deep when it comes to the decisions that caused PeaceHealth to select the Riverbend location for the new hospital.

I have included the responses because they illustrate something I think is unique about the role the local newspaper plays in helping the community engage in on-going political debate. It is clear people in our community enjoy engaging in public discourse—and that the **Register-Guard** enables such dialogue and exchange to take place.)

* * * * * * * *

When I first relocated to Eugene four years ago, I was impressed with the new facility that was preparing to open at the Sacred Heart Medical Center at Riverbend in Springfield.

I had a special fondness for the old facility, now called the University District hospital, because my oldest son was born there when I was in graduate school at the University of Oregon in 1967. I think Sister Monica Heeran was working in the front office when my son was discharged to go home.

I was stunned at the state-of-the art facility developed at RiverBend. One of my first guest viewpoints I wrote for the **Register-Guard** was a piece in which I commended the sisters for having the vision to create a 100-year plan.

I chastised those who felt it was too extravagant. I reminded the critics they should be thankful the hospital was reinvesting local health care profits in the community.

My decades of hospital experience, however, caused me to be suspicious of any plans to keep the old University District hospital open once the RiverBend facility was open and fully operational. It did not make financial sense to spend huge dollars to keep acute care at the aging facility.

I had lunch with Mel Pyne, then the PeaceHealth chief executive officer, and queried him about the plans to renovate the old facility. I had a similar dilemma at the hospital where I had worked in Santa Cruz, California, after we acquired a nearby failing competitor hospital. We chose to use the acquired facility for non-acute inpatient and inpatient and outpatient services, and we consolidated all in-patient services on the main hospital campus.

As I expected, there was a long history of political controversy in which some lobbied strongly that the University District hospital was critical to assuring Eugene residents that they would have access to health care without traveling to RiverBend.

I realized that for emergency care from most parts of Eugene the connection with the RandyPape Beltline provided a direct linkage to RiverBend. I have not seen any studies that show increased risk because of need to be transported to RiverBend instead of University District hospital.

If a financial model were driving the decision of what to do with the University District hospital, the decision would be a no-brainer.

There would be no doubt about the need to do something else with the old site other than resurrecting its ability to continue to provide emergency and acute inpatient care.

It is no coincidence that PeaceHealth once again has asked for an extension on its plans to renovate the old facility. I appreciate the fact that the PeaceHealth University District hospital has a negative 26 percent operating margin, compared with RiverBend' 4.78 percent margin. I realize that PeaceHealth's current financial position is stretching to the point that several top executives have exited from the organization.

The new management team, however tentative until a new CEO can be located, must deal with a reality I suspect few want to confront. They must resist doing the politically correct thing and duplicating acute-inpatient services at the University District facility because of political pressure and do the financially prudent thing by fully integrating all acute inpatient services into the expansive campus at RiverBend, where there is more than sufficient capacity and surrounding space to add services and, as regional demand dictates, increase inpatient bed capacity.

At some time in the future, someone at PeaceHealth is going to have to bite the bullet and confront reality. It does not make any financial sense to operate two acute-care inpatient facilities serving the same service area.

I do not fault those who advocate for the politically correct decision. But I caution those who do to realize that such an action adds significant debt to an organization that already is distressed financially due to a variety of factors, not the least of which is servicing the debt of the new facility and absorbing the expense of maintaining duplicate services at two facilities in the same marketplace.

I am willing to say the unspeakable and raise the politically incorrect subject. I think the community needs to support the notion of not rebuilding an acute-care facility on the old University District site. Find another option that makes sense. Don't duplicate acute inpatient services unnecessarily. It is not in the best interest of the community, even though it may appear to be the politically correct decision.

PeaceHealth at RiverBend is an excellent asset of this community. Don't encumber it with unnecessary debt.

(**NOTE:** The following are the comments that were sent to the newspaper in response to the article. They do a great job of showing the diverse views of a community that is clearly divided over its support of both PeaceHealth and the local city council. They also give a broader perspective on the events that led to the decision to build the new hospital at the RiverBend site.

* * * * * * *

1. *If Kitty and her cronies and all the whiners in Eugene not cried and moaned about losing a hospital downtown then I think PeaceHealth would have taken it down. But Kitty and her old lady cronies of the City Council who ignored the Bethen District and focus all their energy on the University District whole have pulled their heads out and thought for a minute this would not have been a problem.*

2. You are seeing local socialism at its finest. Placing endless obstructions to the hospital when it decided to expand caused them to move to Springfield. Now that Eugene has soiled its nest it cries a hollow whine. Close UDH. The transients will figure out a plan. They always do.

3. Roger—you are correct, of course. This town is run by politically correct idiots. Thus, everything of quality has moved to North Eugene and Springfield. As for the UDH, you can put lipstick on a pig, but it is still a pig. Just the fact that it is an architectural eyesore is enough reason to tear it down.

4. Eugene deserves a mayor named Kitty. . .

5. I live in SE Eugene, and I don't like the thought of having to drive all the way to Springfield for a trip to the emergency room. I know the University location may be expensive to run and an "eyesore," but we have no other hospitals nearby. (Yes, I remember who's "fault" that is!) However, closing the University location would cause a major inconvenience for Eugene area residents.

6. Mr. Hite's opinion is business based, not patient care centered, which is a sad commentary on state of health care in the US. People's lives should not be valued by how much they are costing us. One of PeaceHealth's mission statements is social responsibility. Mr. Hite is right, he is politically incorrect, and it rhymes with social irresponsibility. The comments reflected above show ignorance about the care provided at the University District Hospital. It is also not about convenience, I mean, really, we can't all live right next door to Riverbend! University District has a LOT to offer this community, *people just don't know it. It would be nice to see an article on the good works done by PeaceHealth in this community, especially at University district.*

7. If the University district hospital is really running at a -26% profit margin, i.e., loss, they need to stop that. It means they are hemorrhaging money. It can't go on. It would be interesting to understand why they are losing so much money there. Probably too many people who stiff them. It will be too bad if Eugene loses its downtown emergency operation. Maybe Eugene should have thought more about the consequences when they chased PeachHealth out of town!

8. Eugene's mayor and city council played a high stakes game of chicken with the proposed hospital expansion. They lost, for the citizens of Eugene. They tried to dictate their agenda, none of which had anything to do with health care. It can be modeled this way: Eugene is like the bad-tempered fishwife who has an extreme overabundance of self-esteem. Springfield is like the shy girl with the heart of gold. Eugene's ruling class was so encumbered by its own hubris that it could not see or comprehend that there was a much more attractive option just across the river. Eugene is slowly becoming a moribund enclave of the self-congratulatory glitterati.

9. Don't worry about the trip to Springfield for the ER. EmX will take you! (Don't worry, there's plenty of room on one!) Perhaps the building can be converted to condos, offices, and retail. Oh wait, that would be next to impossible to get approval for that in Eugene. Oh yeah, and there's probably no demand for offices as Eugene historically screws businesses right out of town.

92

Retail? Well, maybe some head shops and tattoo parlors would thrive on the first floor. . . Or how about a parking structure? Oh wait, Eugene hates cars. Scratch that too. Well I guess folks can all move to Springfield to be closer to the hospital, where there's some businesses allowed, and cars are reviled.

10. I recommend some psychiatric counseling. . . The idea that Eugene chased Sacred Wallet out of town is a nice talking point but disconnected from actual facts. Not that facts matter anymore for our polarized, post rational society. I'm not a fan of either "side" in Eugene politics—I think both are deceptive.

Eugene is promoting a quarter billion dollar widening of the Beltline, now is that supposedly hating cars? Eugene and Springfield's city councils are united in supporting the nearly half-billion dollar widening of I-5 through Lane County—an ODOT and Federal decision, but both cities and the counties are in favor of this, too.

The only reason the West Eugene Parkway was not built is the Federal Highway administration realized they'd lose the lawsuit, since it violated every transportation law that applied (dating back to Lyndon Johnson and Richard Nixon).

I'm glad that PeaceHealth spared no expense in their new complex. I hope they are correct that building next to a "river bend" will never, every risk inundation of their center and that the 100 year floods will never happen there again. Just be happy to pay higher health care premiums and bills to pay off the massive debt this new complex required. Eugene and Springfield have an "edifice complex" to spend huge amounts on overbuilt centers (hospitals, sports arenas) while the economy continues to crash. I guess we have our priorities.

11. A little off subject but there's some myths that require a response . . . the WEP was killed off by Kitty herself . . . she very publicly withdrew Eugene's participation in the project despite two voter-approved mandates. And the fools in Eugene reelected her. They get what they deserve. Just like the bums, the downtown, the lack of business, the patchouli-oiled hippies, the transsexual parade (aka the Eugene Celebration.) Some communities serve as a warning to the rest of society.

12. PeaceHealth left Eugene because it was too impatient to work with the Eugene city council. The CEO at that time had a personal vendetta against Eugene and was looking for any reason to abandon a location the hospital had been for nearly 100 years! Making a facility for a projected population was a foolish mistake. It only continues to get worse as they try to compensate for this massive error. The spiteful and flimsy reasons for exiting Eugene will be a burden to PeaceHealth for many years to come.

13. No burden at all as soon as they close down the Eugene hospital cash hemorrhage. Face it, the leaders you elected scre*wed the pooch on this one and all the revisionist history in the world won't change it. Your elected mental midgets could not even find a close in replacement site. Yep, a fine bunch that Eugene brain trust YOU elected (and it a uniquely hilarious Eugene twist, you RE-ELECTED) did. Maybe they should talk to Hugo Chavez, he is their kind of people and he has lots of spare $.s. Oh, sorry, he doesn't. He drove their

economy into the ground. Iike I said, they have lots in common.

14. PeaceHealth was not driven out of Eugene by our all-too-often-too-liberal city council. The council has long been too liberal. But blaming them for the loss of Sacred Heart is a bum rap. It may be widely held fiction but it is fiction nonetheless. PeaceHealth moved to Riverbend, a location that just happened to be located smack dab in the middle of McKenzie Willamette Hospital's most lucrative zip code, because it was the FIRST choice of the corporation's leadership all along. Let me say that again: Not their last choice, their first choice.

A decade ago, PeachHealth was all set to remodel and expand in place. Then one summer McKenzie Willamette announced its own ambitious fundraising and immediate expansion plans. Suddenly, PeaceHealth determined remodeling in place was a terrible idea. They needed to find a new site immediately if not sooner.

By that fall, corporate leaders hastily took several site alternatives to their local advisory board, their senior medical staff, their principal donors and others, recommending Riverbend. The response was uniformly negative. None of those folks wanted to take Eugene's hospital to Springfield.

Publically, the Riverbend site was taken off the table. Most hospital stakeholders were told the land was no longer available. But PeaceHealth, without informing the membership of their local board, formed a special corporation in Washington that cooperated with a new-

ly-arrived local developer who tied up a major portion of the RiverBend land.

The corporation was soon ready to announce (with front page aerial photography) that it would build at north Coburg Road and Crescent Drive . . . on land owned by Wildish, the city itself and the 4J School District.

The only problems were: 1) they did not have their ducks in a row on the land acquisition (e.g. neither the city nor the 4J Board has made a commitment to make their land available); 2) the property was outside the city limits requiring council-approved annexation; and 3), it required a metro plan amendment approved by the elected leaders of Eugene, Springfield and Lane County.

None of these problems was news to senior PeaceHealth management. They must have known their newly announced plan was going to be a tough sell. They knew the council would want to keep the hospital closer to the city center as a centerpiece for downtown redevelopment. In retrospect, it appears they were planning on it.

The developer with the paper interest in the Riverbend parcel led a group of several leading citizens (most of whom were closely affiliated with the hospital's local board, foundations and staff) to anonymously fund a series of political cartoons—on the front page of the Register-Guard—lampooning the city council.

The cartoons were as hard hitting as they were unprecedented and inappropriate. But they carried an element of truth—soundly attacking the council for its

96

actions against the publicly approved West Eugene Parkway. (Even I loved some of them.) The campaign appeared to be one that was always going to be secretly funded. But the cartoons were so shocking to the public's sense of fairness that the identity of those behind it was finally divulged.

Nevertheless, the attacks on the council succeeded. The council capitulated . . . ultimately giving PeaceHealth its way with the Crescent site. But the hospital did not want to win. It wanted Riverbend. By that time the hospital's support groups were ready to take Eugene's hospital to Springfield. The Springfield council, still smarting from losing the federal courthouse to Eugene, was only too happy to cooperate to the max from the get-go.

The only problems with the move have been: 1) financial and regulatory harm was inflicted (many of us believe intentionally so) upon McKenzie Willamette Hospital; 2) the location provides terrible access for a good chunks of Eugene; 3) the location required spending the major part of a decade's worth of this metro area's share of federal and state transportation dollars to improve the Beltline and the Beltline/I-5 interchange; 4) the location is in an especially flood prone area if the up-river dams break; and, 5) the hospital is much too rich for our blood.

The last point, that the hospital is so big and fancy that it is now losing money hand over fist, has accrued despite the fact that it was largely build with hundreds of millions of dollars of debt financed at the lowest possible interest rate by virtue of the use of revenue bonds backed with the full faith and credit of the State of Ore-

gon—a device only available to officially non-profit entities.

Riverbend hospital is a monument not to humble and wise community forethought but to institutional hubris of the worst kind.

One of the political (1.e. regulatory) prices PeaceHealth had to pay for permanently wounding Springfield's other (once genuinely community) hospital was promising to do something significant at the Hilyard campus.

Now PeaceHealth needs to follow through with those University District commitments, no matter how much it may crimp the future expansion plans of its once-public-spirited leadership—or the huge salaries of its remaining senior executives.

15. A lot of revisionist history going on here. Below is the link for the homepage of the Register-Guard for September 8, 2001. Three articles on the front page to read, the lead, and "Hospital picks Springfield" is about PeaceHealth's decision to move to Riverbend, which continues on 10A and includes a timeline. I love this part, "The announcement capped a stormy six months, during which PeaceHealth's plans to build a hospital in north Eugene met with controversy, recriminations and opposition by City Council members and citizen groups. A turning point in PeaceHealth's decision to look to Springfield, Yordy said, came June 27, when the Eugene City Council without warning voted to begin rezoning the north Eugene property to prevent a hospital from going there." The second story entitled, "Officials' responses to decision mixed" documents the Eugene City Council's backpedaling, finger-pointing, and denial of accountability. And the third article, entitled, "Springfield leaders pleased with the deal" pretty much says it all.

16. Interesting. It would be great if the RG would run this summary again. City Council not to blame? The editorial on page 12A should be read too. "But the conventional wisdom was that PeaceHealth's long association with Eugene would prompt the non-profit health organization's officials to look past the council's pedantic, self-righteous inability to grasp the health provider's situation and to find a way to remain in the city."

17. Revisionist? One can only hope/ that the Register-Guard's reporters and the sometimes-publisher-driven editorial page brought the PeaceHealth line on who was to blame does not make it so. Nothing just mentioned here speaks to the hospital's original intent . . . which was Riverbend. And the city council did in the end completely capitulate. A lot of things happened after Yordy's magical decision date. He chose to ignore them and the press failed to report them. Many of us were so unhappy with our city council—and for good reasons—that we did not see what was really going on. . . .the furthering of PeaceHealth's near perfect monopoly in local and regional health care delivery and the removal of hundreds of jobs out of the metro area.

More recently, PeaceHealth has determined to move much of its support staff from Springfield to Vancouver, WA. Is the Eugene City Council responsible for that, too? No. It is just our nine-hundred-pound gorilla/enemy-of-the-people doing its own thing.

18.   PeaceHealth is the "enemy-of-the-people"?   Really?   That makes it pretty hard to take seriously anything you previously wrote.   Sounds like you have an axe to grind.

19.   Comment #15 is how I remember it.   Whatever PeaceHealth's inner wishes—I'm not a mind reader— the City of Eugene and several of the city's denizens did their utmost to make sure PeaceHealth didn't build in Eugene.   My recollection: they wanted to build off Coburg Road, and Eugene did everything to prevent it. (No, they weren't going to expand in the campus area; that would have meant driving out blocks and blocks of people, who rightly stopped any possibility of that.)   A lot of comments are typical of a very odd mindset in Eugene; a valuable institution (PeaceHealth or UO or a prospective HP plant) is cast as the enemy of the people.   Fortunately, UO can't be forced out!

20.   One angle on this story that was never reported: as the PeaceHealth vs. McKenzie battle was unfolding, Dave F. and the UO were quietly building support for a takeover of the university building, turning it into a teaching hospital and launching a full-blown medical school at the Eugene campus.   This was shot-down by supporters of OHSU, and PeaceHealth was left to play a cynical game of applying for permits for university hospital beds it knew it didn't need of want.

Also a correction to laying the blame for WEP at Kitty's feet.   It took two votes on the PC to kill WEP and Kitty brought along her lap dog Alan Zelenka to provide the key second "no" vote.   Eugene is now saddled with two depressing and ugly facilities owned by PeaceHealth. I'm really surprised that PH hasn't been forced to pull the plug on the university site.   It's like the walking wounded over there, but that pretty much describes most of Eugene anyway, so you know, you get what you vote for.

21. Lots of speculation here, and lots of facts and issues still ignored and unexplained. One neglected factor is that if the university site closes, that leaves a market vacuum in Eugene, and opportunity that a well-capitalized for-profit company will probably not neglect. Any system or corporate acquisition of a hospital niche is extremely valuable in a world where the only survivors will be those systems/corporations who are too big to fail. PeaceHealth has recently abandoned some markets, and has suffered some defections. It would probably be unwise for them to vacate Eugene completely. It would certainly not be good for Eugene—and not only for reason of convenience. If you think PeaceHealth is the ultimate in money-grubbing, you haven't lived in a market where the for-profits rule the roost.

22. From the general tone of the comments here—and on practically every other RG article—you would think Eugene/Springfield were a POW Camp forcibly imprisoning all of its residents in a hellhole. If Eugene is such a horrible place, with decaying everything and dishonest politicians and disastrously bad decision-making and class warfare between "the people" and big scary institutions, why do you all still live here?? Mr. Hite says that keeping the University District facility open is "politically correct." Why? I don't understand this assertion. Some commenter's claim that they are inconvenienced by having to go to Springfield for the hospital. When is the last time you drove to the University? I live near the Whitaker and it takes me less time to get to Gateway than to get to the UO. The only people inconvenienced by this are people who live immediately adjacent to the University.

23.   Eugene is now saddled with two "ugly" PeaceHealth sites solely because PeaceHealth refused to expand at either one. PeaceHealth was perfectly content with their plans to remodel and expand in-place on Hilyard—until days and weeks after McKenzie Willamette announced its intent to do a major expansion to its facilities and services.

Then, those "dumb" liberals in Eugene wanted the hospital to expand at the Willamette site rather than moving to the edge of the metro area.   Had PeaceHealth taken either course, Eugene would not be saddled with two "ugly" underused sites . . . and Springfield would have a stronger, still-community-owned hospital.

And PeaceHealth would not be stuck with a big fancy Riverbend monument to its excessive corporate aspirations—one it now whines (through this op ed writer) that it cannot afford—despite using hundreds of millions of low-interest funds borrowed under the name of the State of Oregon. But, of course, that is the price they have to pay for landing at a huge site where they hoped (judging by their own public statements) and still hope to control everything that is build right around them for the next hundred years.   In this community tragedy, the dumb bodies are buried all over the place—not just at the Eugene City Hall.

(Postscript: On Tuesday, September 13, 2011, the **Register-Guard** continued the dialogue over the hospital plans for the University District Hospital by publishing a follow-up op-ed piece in which a local investor advocated for creating a new partnership between the OU and PeaceHealth for a medical program at the university and a conversion of the site to a medical school affiliation agreement. I suspect that for the foreseeable future my initial op ed piece should be credited with bringing the public-debate to the forefront of local politics.

19

"Left on the Cutting Room Floor"

(**NOTE:** The essays that follow represent all of the articles I have written and submitted over the past three years that were not published by the **Register-Guard.** I respect the editorial judgment of Jack Wilson and I am confident there were good reasons to pass on publishing these opinions. I always feel good that each is given a serious consideration—and in light of the many that have been published, I never feel slighted with an article is passed over.

In retrospect, I can see in each case, at least one or two good reasons why the editorial may not have met Mr. Wilson critical standard. As you will see, in the final analysis, he may have protected me from myself and sheltered me from unwarranted public criticism.

I consider the creating of an editorial opinion essay an art in itself. I enjoy taking the time to put my ideas into the form necessary for submission.

The nice thing about this collection is that I have a vehicle, much more limited than the 60,000 readers of the **Register-Guard,** however, that allows me to share my ideas and opinions.

* * * * * * *

"Beyond Profitability"

(**Note:** The following submission was the initial editorial I submitted a couple of days before the article that obviously re-opened old wounds about the stalled-plans for revising the University District PeaceHealth facility. I was personally more interested in having readers better understand the subject of productivity management and its impact on hospital quality.

* * * * * * * *

I was not surprised by the comparisons made in the two excellent front-page **Register-Guard** stories about the financial challenges facing both Eugene/Springfield area hospitals.

I do take exception, however, to one observation made by an analyst working for RBC Capital who was quoted as saying, *"For-profit hospitals typically perform better financially than non-profits [because] non-profits operate on a different model, and they typically get by through donations and endowments."*

A lot of not-for-profit hospitals—including my former employer in Santa Cruz—Dominican Hospital—contradicts such old-school conventional wisdom. It is a similar size to RiverBend—yet it posted net operating revenues in excess of $35 million this past year! In recent years the blur between management styles of either type of hospital has come into focus. There is nothing significantly different between the two types of owner-ship. For both hospital models, productivity management overshadows all other issues. Improve productivity and you improve profitability. Given this new Conventional Wisdom in health care management, it is time to ask: *Where does the profitability slope intersect the quality slope in the graphing of the health care equation?*

I don't want to deprecate anyone interested in helping the general public learn how to understand health care finances. However, it is understandably hard for an average person to appreciate the magnitude of dollars associated with running a multi-million dollar business like a general acute care hospital. It is easy to be overly impressed with the magnitude of dollars. The **Register-Guard** reported did a good job of addressing such a problem by putting the magnitude of charitable care in proper perspective.

The important comparison was not the total dollars McKenzie-Willamette Medical Center expended on charity care--$1.47 million dollars. But the fact it is slightly more than a half-of-one-percent of its $255 million dollars of patient revenue. And, given the fact that McKenzie-Willamette Medical Center pays taxes, one should expect PeaceHealth—which enjoys tax-exempt status in exchange for its not-for-profit status—would rightfully shoulder a bigger cost hit to its operating expenses--$28 million or 3.2 percent of its $873 million in patient revenues. It was also useful to point out the difference between totaling up uncompensated "sticker price" bills versus the true cost of providing such services—reminding us nobody pays full sticker price.

If we had a single-payer national health program, "charity care" contributions by either for-profit or not-for-profit hospitals would become an obsolete, irrelevant statistic. But given our broken national system that still depends on cost-shifting, hospitals must continue to focus on managing payer-mix.

In the article focused on McKenzie-Willamette hospital, we learn the hospital has been successful in managing its "payer-mix." 56.8 percent of McKenzie-Willamette's patients have insurance, compared with RiverBend where their patient mix only contains 31.5 percent insured; and, the University District where only 26.7 percent of its patients are insured.

Marketing a hospital to the insured patients through contracting with HMO's and managed care patients isn't a strategy deployed only by for-profit hospitals, as one analyst quoted in the **Register-Guard** story suggests. It is a strategy ALL hospitals—including PeaceHealth—must deploy.

PeaceHealth and McKenzie both receive the same reimbursement for Medicare and Medicaid patient segments of their "payer-mix." The size of the privately insured segment of the hospital's business is the foundation upon which hospitals cost-shift the shortfall that comes from government sponsored patients as well as non-paying patients.

In the McKenzie focused article, the statement is made that the hospital's financial performance reflects *"responsible hospital management practices—keeping a lid on costs without jeopardizing quality."*

And, there's the rub! How do we know the focus on "productivity management" doesn't get to the point where it impacts quality? At some point the slope of improving productivity and profitability intersects the slope of quality—and as productivity and profitability increases, quality declines.

McKenzie-Willamette had an operating margin of 7.04 percent last year, compared with a 4.78 percent at Sacred Heart Riverbend; and, a striking NEGATIVE 26 percent at the University District facility. How much margin is enough? What are the quality metric indicators we as consumers should be aware of that will make us feel comfortable that productivity improvement and profitability are not being obtained at the expense of quality?

As a former hospital administrator who is now several years removed from the task of being constantly attuned to a hospital financial balance sheet and its monthly operational "profit and loss" statement, I realize all hospitals must earn "excess revenue over expenses (EROE)" if they wish to maintain financial viability and have resources to re-invest back into operations.

(After a recent visit to Santa Cruz where I listened to staff at my former hospital lament the pressure and stress, I wonder if $35 million EROE is too much? I wonder if they are approaching or have surpassed the point of intersect? I wonder, too, how does one factor "stress" into the quality equation?)

Given the fact that virtually half of a hospital's annual operating budget is spent on labor, it is understandable that all hospitals—regardless of their ownership—must attend to managing "productivity." As we look for the appropriate quality metrics it will be necessary, but not sufficient, to identify the medical outcome metrics. We also need to look at the metrics that measure the quality of the workplace and its staff well-being. While it was interesting to see the financial comparisons between McKenzie-Willamette and the PeaceHealth facilities, I would like to see a future article focus on what should be the most important consumer concern—namely, the key quality metrics that measures clinical outcomes as well as care-giver satisfaction and well-being.

20

"Just say No to Drugs—Commercials about Viagra and Cialis"

I enjoy watching 60 Minutes. It challenges me to think about what I believe regarding the major social, political, and economic challenges of our times. However, my favorite element in each program is always the ending five-minute social commentary by Andy Rooney.

Drug companies who make Viagra and Cialis advertise on 60 Minutes. That means I will probably never see or hear Andy Rooney rail against such ads. So, in the spirit of Andy, I offer this editorial observation.

I am not a media censor. I respect a company's right to buy advertisement in the newspaper and on the air as long as it conforms to common sense standards of taste and decency.

What concerns me about the Calais and Viagra commercials has nothing to do with the way the ads are portrayed—it has to do with the message the frequency of the ads send to a whole generation of youth.

Those who determine the political correctness of television commercials—and what type of ads to accept or reject—should revisit their standards. Specifically, somebody needs to re-write the rules for direct advertising of prescription drugs. It is a very lucrative strategy for the pharmaceutical companies to have patients pressure physicians into prescribing drugs. Viagra and Cialis are a great case in point. It is far more effective than relying on drug detail representatives to make their rounds to physician offices with drug samples.

I can't believe I am the only male in America who has become absolutely tired and annoyed at the constant airing of the Cialis and Viagra commercials. I am offended by the false image the ads create about the American male's hierarchy of concerns.

It isn't like the commercials air occasionally. They are clearly one of the most prominent advertisers of our current times. And I object. I'm not a prude. I'm not a self-righteous moralist. I just don't like the false conclusion one can draw about American culture and about what American men are concerned about.

Consider this the beginning of my official campaign against the advertisement of Cialis and Viagra. I am tired of the message such TV commercials project to current and future generations of men.

What do mothers and fathers say to their young ones who innocently ask, "What is erectile dysfunction?"

I wonder, too, what does a parent says when a child asks, "Why should you be worried about getting an erection that last longer than four hours!"

But that's the problem with raising such concerns into the social awareness of the American marketplace. It demands an explanation. It is too bad Andy Rooney can't address the issue!

There are certain things in human relationship that are best left to the privacy of intimate sexual relationships—and in confidential conversations with one's physician. It may well be the case that some men long for the fountain of youth in their sexuality. If you have a problem, discuss it with your physician. We don't need to discuss it in the marketplace.

I know there are young men in our society who think relationships are all about virility. How are we going to teach them about true relationships when they are bombarded with ads that emphasize men worry about being ready for the right moment with their erections!

In looking back on my earlier days, I can see the problems many men faced were problems created because they could get an erection! But that is an altogether different social problem many men spend a lifetime learning to manage!

I was the son of a father who never educated me about such things as the problems created by erectile dysfunction—I don't know if it such a condition ever existed in the Greatest Generation. Maybe it is the exclusive product of the "Me generation?"

Let's stop this exploitation of masculinity. Take the erectile dysfunction ads out of the media marketplace vocabulary—keep it in the confidential dialogue between patient and physician.

There, Andy Rooney, now you owe me one!

21

A "Flashbulb Moment" A Decade Ago this 9/11

Bob Welch uses the term "flashbulb moment" to describe the handful of events that time etches forever in the archives of our memories.

September 11, 2001 was for everyone a flashbulb moment.

Like most Americans, I still recall vividly where I was and what I was doing on that tragic moment of American history. Sharing such personal recollections reminder us of how history binds us together in ways that strengthen our shared heritage as Americans.

My wife Debby and I were traveling in Europe with my mother-in-law Verla. We were staying in a modest, no-frills hotel that was within walking distance to the famous Glockenspiel clock tower in Munich, Germany—it was the first evening of a two-week summer vacation.

We returned to our room after a traditional German dinner of bratwurst and beer while enjoying the brass band festivities at the Hofbrau House. I turned on the television, only to watch in disbelief as two jets collided with the world trade center towers in New York City!

It was early morning on 9/11 in New York—and late evening in Munich.

Once we realized we weren't watching a b-grade horror-film, we rushed down the narrow hotel corridor to Deb's mom room. We pounded on the door and in the confusion caused mom to actually lock instead of unlock her door! When we finally got her to our room we all sat down and looked at each other, frightened and feeling terribly isolated—several thousand miles from home. And to make matters even more disconcerting, we were staying in a hotel that was smack-dab in the middle of a Muslim section of Munich!

For the duration of our trip I realized how large the Muslim influence had become in Europe—especially in Switzerland. I was paranoid every time I saw traditional Muslim clothing on women and dark-skinned Muslim men—and kept telling myself that 99.9% of Muslims are peace-loving and God-worshipping humans. I had not given a lot of thought to the Muslim presence in America until that "flashbulb moment" of 9/11.

I was surprised at my own almost "cowardly" response. I felt terribly alone and vulnerable—an American in a hostile world. My immediate reaction was to pack up and head back to America on the first plane we could catch the next morning! Deb was more practical—she recognized what would prove to be true—that it would be virtually impossible to catch a plane for several days—even if we resolved to scrap the vacation and head for home!

In contrast to me, Deb wanted to get an American flag and proudly wear it on her sweater so everyone could see she wasn't intimidated to be out and about in the new world reality of the 9/11 atrocity!

The next day we continued with our tour plans. Complete strangers came up to us, almost in tears, expressing their shared grief over what had happened to America. The only contrast to this genuine compassion and sympathy was a cynical remark made by one insensitive Munich cab driver who scoffed and volunteered his opinion about the tragedy, indicating how it served America right for its arrogant treatment of the rest of the world!

The insensitive cab driver's comments were indelibly captured in my 9/11 flashbulb moment. I thought a lot about his remark during the two-weeks of our trip—granted, he was a middle-eastern man living in Munich—a city devastated by American and its allies during an earlier war—but a city that reminds us old enemies can become friends. I am an optimist and look forward to a time when nobody looks upon American as an enemy, or a country deserving to be targeted for terrorist killings.

Many of the Europeans we met were anxious about how the wounded Americans would react to the atrocity. How would they fight a war against a terrorist organization that had no geographic boundaries, no standing army—how could America's most powerful military fight against such an elusive enemy?

I remember how uncomfortable I was for the balance of our trip as we made our way through Austria, Switzerland, and ended up in Paris for our return trip home.

Sadly, my flashbulb moment caused me to become irrationally suspicious of Muslims—a perspective I struggle with today. I am learning to have much greater sympathy for American Muslims who do not deserve to be viewed with such prejudice. I recall my own immediate fears in the aftermath of 9/11 to realize how such views are formed—and how difficult they are to keep in check!

When we landed in San Francisco, I had a lump in my throat as I looked out at the Golden Gate Bridge. The flashbulb moment of 9/11 awakened in me a new sense of pride and patriotism. In the weeks and months after 9/11 I was proud of how America picked itself up and worked together to clear away the rubble of the ground-zero-site in Manhattan.

I recently watched with pride the television tour anchorman Matt Lauer broadcast as he accompanied a construction foreman up to the 78th floor of the new trade center tower being built at the rate of about a floor a week by impassioned American workers determined to complete the final thirty floors and bring a new building to replace one of the two lost towers.

I was glad, too, that a decade later, American soldiers settled the score with the architect of that terrible event.

On this ten-year anniversary of 9/11 I hope all Americans will pause and share with each other their memory of that "flashbulb moment" in American history and make sure we never forget people who lost their lives and the brave firefighters and police who arrived as first-responders. Let's all celebrate what binds us together as Americans, regardless of our ethnic origins or our religious beliefs.

22

"The Reality of a Maxed-Out Federal Credit Card"

In my book **I Still Buy Green Bananas: Reflections on Living and Dying in our Culture of Denial,** (amazon.com, 2010), I illustrated the concept of *a culture of denial* by describing how such a belief structure allows our government to avoid thinking about its own mortality. Like so many Americans indulging in credit-card enabled "instant gratification" our federal government is living in a culture of denial.

As Congress debates the conditions under which we should raise the credit limit on our national credit card we need to come to terms with the mythology of our nation's sense of financial immortality.

When attorneys invented the concept of a *corporation*, there was an unintended consequence of such a brilliant financial tool. On the positive side, a corporation allowed a mom-and-pop business to transcend the life-span of the company's founders and create a legal surrogate responsible for all the debts and liabilities of the business independent of its founders. This allowed the business to pass forward in time debts and assets. It enables investors to own something that could transcend the life-span of a mere mortal.

Our culture of denial was further enabled by the creation of the ubiquitous credit card. No longer did humans have to pay-as-you-go. The credit card was the great enabler of our desire for instant gratification. It enabled us to deny the reality of what we could afford because it pushed forward in time the consequences of debt and allowed us to enjoy the moment.

The unintended consequences of the *corporation* concept and the idea of a credit-card with no limit is that these instruments allowed our government to perpetuate the myth of its own "immortality." In the real world we deal with the fact a human life is finite. Death is what gives value to each day and causes us to realize the consequences of our personal decisions. A government can thrive in a culture of denial because it enjoys the myth it will live forever.

In the long run death is also a reality for governments— it is not a matter of **if**, it is a matter of **when**. Given such a reality we should wish to have a government that enjoys good health and lives as long as possible. Huge debt, however, is like a malignant cancer that will hasten the demise of any government before its time.

It is quite easy to illustrate how humans would behave if they knew they were going to live forever. Would you pay down your mortgage? Would you limit your credit card debt? Would you not indulge yourself in instant gratification? After all, you would have forever to pay off your debt!

Humans know they are mortal and accountable for the consequences of their decisions. Why is it that we don't hold our government accountable for such behavior as well? How do we come to terms with the fact that the government debt is actually **our** debt? Each American household's share is over $100 thousand dollars; our individual share of national debt is approximately $40 thousand dollars! What would a financial advisor tell us if we were dealing with such a condition in our personal lives? Why are we unwilling to confront our government with the same harsh advice?

Imagine what would happen if we acknowledged our government is not immortal? Imagine if we felt vulnerable for the consequences of our immediate financial decisions instead of passing them forward? Perhaps we would delay expensive "wants" and pork-barrel projects and focus on basic "needs?" Perhaps we would start "saving" and developing a "rainy-day fund" so we could be prepared for the unexpected. Perhaps we would deny ourselves things because we couldn't afford them instead of enjoying the "instant gratification" that accompanies the mythology a federal credit card can never be maxed-out.

Sadly, the world financial situation today is evidence of how the cultural of denial mythology impacts governments. Europe is replete with many so-called immortal governments that are on the verge of collapse. Greece is probably going to avoid financial death for the time being because it will be rescued by the life-support of other European financial partners—but many of those rescuing Greece are also confronting the reality of their own financial "mortality."

Our finite human life is the perfect condition because of—not in spite of—the fact it ends in death! Perhaps it is time for our government to come to terms with our culture of denial and realize that governments, too, are mortal and finite. Hopefully the life of the American government will be long and prosperous, but it is folly and hubris to believe any government is immortal.

The more we buy into a culture of denial, the easier it is for our government to behave irresponsibly and to pass forward the consequences of poor decisions. It is time to wake up and start living within our means and paying down our massive debt. That is what we would do as financially responsible individuals; it is what we should expect of our government as well!

I believe there is a lot of life left in the American government if we start treating the cancer that is killing it.

23

"We are all Victims of Health-Care Cost Shifting"

B ob Welch did an excellent job of researching and reporting the issues contributing to the shocking $1630 dollar invoice Mrs. Leslie Comar received for simply transporting her insulin-dependent son from Autzen stadium a mile and a half to the hospital via ambulance. Mr. Welch's article under-scores one of the biggest challenges of restructuring health care financing. Cost-shifting has got to be elimi-nated. It is a double tax on every health-care consumer and allows the government to effectively avoid paying its fair-share of health care costs.

Few of us, fortunately, receive Mrs. Comar's ambu-lance bill. Make no mistake—like Mrs. Comar most of us receive a hidden cost-shift double-tax each month when we pay our private health insurance bill. It is not an exaggeration to say that the $800 dollar health care bill we pay for my wife's private insurance could be reduced by a minimum of a hundred and fifty dollars each month if it were not for cost shifting. That's an annual additional tax of $1800 each year—slightly more than the single tax levied on Mrs. Comar through her ambulance experience.

Forty years ago the government had an arrangement with providers so they were paid cost-plus for all services purchased by the government for people covered by the Medicare entitlement program. At that time health care was less than 6% of the GDP.

An apocryphal story that best illustrated the hazard of such reimbursement was told about the hospital president who was considering buying a new CAT scanner at a cost of $1 million dollars. He called his controller and asked if such a piece of equipment was covered under the cost-plus Medicare reimbursement rules of the time. If it was, then 50% of the cost would be paid by the government because 50% of the hospital's inpatients were Medicare patients. The controller verified it was covered. "Good," the administrator said, "Then let's buy two!"

Sadly, all health care reimbursement system will be vulnerable to being gamed by folks determined to maximize the system to serve different agendas. The most ubiquitous game over the years has been the strategy of cost-shifting.

I do not advocate a return to cost-plus financing of health care—as it had its share of problems that contributed to waste and inefficiencies in the health care sector of our economy. I do believe, though, that as we move toward deploying an effective national health care system we will need to return to some modified form of uniform payment not based on market leverage, volume purchase discounts, or artificial price structures created by government panels.

I hope that as we deploy health care reform legislation and create quasi-private insurance purchasing cooperatives we do not create another insurance option upon which to unload government shortfalls. The history of health care financing over the past several decades might be characterized as a contest between government, insurance companies, and providers. When the health care GDP climbed toward 10% concerned government regulators tried several schemes to control costs—none produced results that eliminated cost-shifting.

Cost-shifting is a survival strategy for providers who have no other choices because the current financing system is broken. Don't blame the providers who use it. Blame the government that created the system. Hold the government responsible for remedying the situation.

Welch's research pointed out that in Lane County the ambulance cost-shift is born by about 17% of those who paid the $1630 dollars. The other 83% paid less and many examples were provided where a few "frequent flyers" consumed hundreds of thousands of dollars in uncompensated ambulance transportation costs.

Mrs. Comar's example is one of the best arguments for moving toward a single-payer public option. Fundamental to a successful public option is the elimination of cost shifting. The government becomes responsible for paying the costs associated with providing basic health care coverage to all. I was pleased to read that 25% of the people in Lane County pay the $65 dollars a year into the FireMed program so they can avoid the situation faced by Mrs. Comar. It is an example of a voluntary taxation.

Extend the example of voluntary taxing for ambulance coverage and apply the logic to the full range of services we want to be part of our national health care program. Tax people once for paying the true costs associated with government sponsored patients. Charge all users the same fee.

How will we know when we are moving in the right direction with whatever happens on the horizon with our national health care reform legislation? When everybody—private individuals, insurance companies, and government program—all pay the same price for an ambulance trip—a price based on the true costs and reasonable profit-margin for providing the service. Imagine if such a pricing strategy were applied to all other inpatient and outpatient services and procedures.

When cost-shifting is eliminated, that is not the end of our problems. We will still have an inefficient, costly, duplicative health care system that will need rational oversight of the costs and benefits of the health care we provide our citizens.

I agree with Mrs. Comar. She should not have to pay the $1630 dollars. But guess what, Mrs. Comar is not along. Each of us pays annual taxes and then pay an inflated costs for a private health insurance plan we receiving each month. Whether we realize it or not, we are just like Mrs. Comar. Our government continues to present us with a cost-shifted double-tax bill for our broken American health care delivery system. It's time to eliminate cost-shifting.

24

Putting a New Limit on the Nation's Credit Card

I had a strong reaction to the editorial opinion published in the Register-Guard Sunday July 17h by Professor Helen Popper—associate professor of economics at Santa Clara University. Her article cautioned readers about supporting a Constitutional Amendment to require a balanced budget.

I don't know if such an amendment is the solution—or how difficult it would be to enact! But my reaction to her perspective was that she was off-target in focusing on the federal budget; the issue is our nation's credit-card limit!

I had mixed feelings about the perspective Professor Popper used in comparing the debt management of an individual family with the debt management of the federal government. Family credit-card debt has its own mortality—and it is time to affirm the same reality for our government.

My criticism of Popper's perspective is that she makes her point by comparing the importance of debt in a family and used it to support the case that a similar logic applies to our federal government's debt. The government may be generally likened to a family in the sense it must deal with choices to assume debt—but if we are going to make such analog comparisons we need to look critically at how the government is different from an individual family unit. We also need to look at another analogy that makes such a comparison more relevant.

Families are different than governments. Families are mortal and have a life-cycle in which they must grow and take on debt so they can build and develop. Ideally, a successful family meets its debt obligations, accrues wealth, pays down its debt, and in the years of retirement enjoys a debt-free existence where one draws from savings and pensions and social security entitlement and if there is something left over, it is passed on to future generations.

Yes, such a family debt-management cycle is becoming far less a reality for more and more families as they struggle in today's economy and deal with massive credit-card debt management! And, of course, such a debt-free future has disappeared for our nation as we have accrued over $40,000 dollars of long-range debt for ever American!

Governments, however, are entities that perceive themselves as exempt from the rules governing debt for mere mortals. The government can and does take on a different kind of debt—a debt that transcends the lifetime individual humans and families.

It isn't about the fact both families and government need to manage debt. The problem is that the government—like any responsible family unit—should not have access to a credit card that has no limit. It doesn't make sense for a family and it doesn't make sense for a government—but for significantly different reasons.

To illustrate my point, what incentives would an individual family have to pay off a mortgage or a debt if it knew it could simply pass the obligation forward indefinitely? Why pay off the balance of any credit card? Why not enjoy instant gratification and purchase anything one desired? That is the sad state of affairs we find with our current government appetite for charging now and passing debt obligation forward as though the government is immortal when it comes to credit debt.

I am not an economist—but I am someone who is always cautious when it comes to critical thinking. Professor Popper is far more qualified that I am to comment on our current national economic picture. But I don't think her argument contributed much enlightenment to the current credit problem.

If you were to ask me if I am in favor of putting a limit on the national credit card I would say "absolutely." Do I balk at realizing it must be raised beyond its current limits? Sure. And it goes without saying I would like this to be the last time we increase the limit.

If you asked me, however, "what should that limit be?" I don't have any sophisticated answer. That will clearly be the source of much heated debate as we approach the drop dead date of August 2, 2011! We must raise the limit, but we must also find ways to limit future spending. In a family setting, we would sort between the "wants" and the "needs."

We know that since the creation of our credit-card driven economy we have developed individual habits of indulging in instant gratification instead of saving and paying as we go along. Such a credit-card mentality makes it difficult to educate future generation of family households from developing good credit management habits. The *"buy now pay later"* mentality has thoroughly infected the spending mentality of Congress.

I don't disagree with Professor Popper's conclusion that we don't always have to have a balanced budget—or with her conclusion that balancing a budget in hard times could make downturn worse.

I can't argue with her hypothesis that a balanced budget amendment doesn't put any obligation on Congress to manage spending during good times. I am among those who want significant cuts in spending and in getting the greatest value for what we spend.

Dr. Popper is off target in comparing family economics with government economics. Government is a "corporation" that has a lifespan that transcends the mere mortality of a human life and an individual family's economy.

Unlike a family economy where responsible couples develop a financial plan designed to pay down debt and leave the family debt free during its retirement years, the government can postpone worrying about debt because it suffers from the illusion it is immortal. It is time to hold our government accountable for its own credit-card mortality! Make this the last increase in our national credit-card limit—and focus on living within our means as a government! You, know, like we are on the same page economically as a national family!

25

"Players Should Stop Being Cheerleaders"

Football players are among the worst offenders—followed by soccer players. Sports fans know what I mean—on-field celebrations! It has become at its best institutionalized immature behavior—at its worst, offensive, taunting and unbecoming behavior. Players are players and cheerleaders are cheerleaders. Stop confusing the roles!

Even in the professional sports arena, the referees have drawn the line with the foolish antics of end-zone dances, belly-bumping celebrations, and border-line taunting behavior of an opposing team. It now seems normative for players to engage in such self-aggrandizing display. Occasionally the celebration is so obnoxious and excessive a referee will toss a flag and penalize a team with a 15 yard assessment on the ensuing kick-off.

Sadly, professional sports teams are exclusively about winning and owners seem willing to over-look the unbecoming behavior of its prima donna athletes—e.g. Terrell Owens. Professional football players represent, after all, the very best of university- trained athletes. So if we are going to abolish such behavior at the professional level we have to go to the source of the problem—the training grounds of the university gridiron.

University sports must assume the responsibility of changing the norm. If they do, then the few athletes who make it to the professional ranks will have experienced four years of non-celebrative discipline. They will have learned to let their playing, not their chest thumping antics shape their images. From this fan's viewpoint, it will enhance, not detract from the excitement of the contest.

Whether we like it or not, the image of university and professional athletes shape the way young high school athletes behave on the playing field. They can and do emulate what they see as their role models. Go to a pop-Warner football game and see how much the norm of celebration is emulated by young boys! Is it any wonder they come into high school and feel such behavior is expected?

Such a reality is sufficient reason for rule-makers in all university football conferences throughout the country to take a stand. Say "No" to any overt display of celebration on the playing field. Make the norm simply setting the ball on the end-zone turn and returning to your team's sideline. Celebrate among teammates with side-line high-fives and bottom slaps. Set the rule so it can be enforced by coaches. They will get the picture and pass it on to their athletes. Any on-field overt display will result in a fifteen-yard penalty assessed on the ensuing kickoff. A second offense will result in the person penalized for end-zone or other on-field individual celebration to have to sit out a segment of the game for a pre-determined period.

It should be the responsibility of university sports programs to eliminate the childish and immature celebrations that take place on the playing field—and

I'm not just talking about what happens in the end-zone after a touchdown.

Coaches should be required to discipline their players to stop the chest-thumping and bumping bravado. Penalize a player who makes gestures or howls like an animal at the moon after they execute a bone-jarring block or tackle. It doesn't add anything positive to their image as an aggressive competitor. It is an overt display of immaturity.

Most football programs take pride is teaching their athletes discipline. It is what enables the individual players to do their part in helping the team successfully execute on both sides of the line of scrimmage. Resisting celebration must become a discipline.

When a team is successful the results speak for themselves. An individual who carries the ball across the goal line is enabled by the effective play of ten other teammates. Everybody on the team has a right to feel proud of the team's achievement. Perhaps that's why defensive players who don't do a lot of scoring have taken it upon themselves to celebrate with chest-thumping antics and gestures after they do what they are supposed to do and successfully thwart an offense play.

It seems like many coaches allow players to confuse their player role with the cheerleader role. When did defensive players decide it was their responsibility to wave their arms and encourage the crowd of spectators to make more noise? Focus on the game and let the fans do what they do. Let the cheerleaders on the sidelines entertain the crowd and lead them in cheers. Let the players play the game.

Imagine what a game would be like if the team focused on its team discipline. Imagine if after a play the defensive players extended their hand and helped up the player they had just successfully stopped for no gain. I am always proud of my team when I see such sportsman-like behavior.

It all comes down to discipline, respect, and positive self-image. The kinds of celebrations we often see after a play or a score represent "in your face" disrespect for an opponent. Many displays of exuberance are forms of taunting.

It is unfortunate, but given the lack of direction by the league and the coaches, many players have come to think that excessive celebration is a player's entitlement. It's time that players stop trying to become cheerleaders.

26

"Presidential Material"

As the Presidential election campaigning season approaches and candidates announce they are putting together an "exploratory committee" to assess support for entering the race, I have strong opinions about what I would like to happen. I believe our political process puts the proverbial cart before the horse. Both parties need to do some homework before we open up the process for applicants.

I take a deep breath and pause when I hear the names Sarah Palin, Donald Trump, Mike Huckabee, Mitt Romney, and scores of lesser know names testing whether they have enough support to warrant launching a serious and expensive Presidential campaign.

My question is not whether these people are qualified to fill the position—but whether we as an electorate have any consensus on what we are seeking? I have not yet decided who I will support—the incumbent or the challenger. I have made up my mind, however, to develop a score card for evaluating the candidates based upon some criteria other than popularity or electability—or on the basis of who makes the most attractive campaign promises. I encourage both political parties to do likewise.

In private industry any large corporation would draft a job description outlining the minimum qualifications for applicants. The description would list specific experiences and background the business wants to know before granting an applicant an interview—e.g., advancing to the presidential primary evaluation period.

If I could tweak our democratic process I would have the two major political parties formulate their own "search committee" before we open the process for "unsolicited" applicants from a wide array of aspiring candidates. Each party should write a job description stating what they are seeking. The criteria should be made public to assist the electorate compare the qualifications of candidates. Candidates should view the Presidential Primary race as the forum in which to demonstrate to the American public---the stockholders in our Democracy--how well they meet their political party's specific criteria.

I know one can argue the US Constitution stipulates the minimum Presidential qualifications: Applicants must be a natural born American citizen who is over the age of 35. The applicant must agree to support the values and governmental rules contained in the US Constitution. That's the description in a nut shell.

It doesn't say "political experience desired" or required. The applicant doesn't have to show a minimum of X years in the US Congress—either the House of Representatives or the US Senate. We don't require any level of education—not even graduation from an accredited college or university. We don't require any law degree. We don't ask applicants to demonstrate evidence of understanding business and economics—or have any business experience even though they are expected to oversee the largest business enterprise in the free world. Sadly, many candidates simply tout whether they know how to work the system to get elected—not whether they are the best qualified to serve once elected.

Without a thoughtful job description that identifies specific qualifications needed by applicants   at this moment in our history we rely upon such things as "media appeal" and "personal charisma" and appeal to a particular ethnic segment of the voting population. I don't mean to imply these are not real considerations, but what is it we really need now in the pool of applicants?

Over the years there have been many unspoken criteria that de facto screened-out qualified would-be Presidential applicants. There was no sign in the government's window that said "Whites Only," or "Catholic Irish Need not Apply," or "No Women Need Apply"—but these criteria certainly were political realities we had to overcome in defining modern "Presidential Material."
Surely we are sophisticated enough in our two-party system to articulate the ideal qualifications and experience we are seeking in our quest for a President in the election of 2012.

The incumbent's party should huddle and define what it wants for the incumbent to continue in his role. Once the party has clearly stated its needs, then the party verifies it endorses the incumbent. It then becomes the task of the incumbent in the campaign process to demonstrate how well he meets his party's expectations as measured by the criteria of their job description. Even though it is considered politically incorrect for an applicant in one's own party to challenge the incumbent, if in fact someone within the incumbent's party demonstrates they better meet the party's criteria, then they deserve to make their case in the Presidential primary. We need to abandon the conventional wisdom of the incumbent being de facto the candidate of choice for the party.

I intend to sit down and write out specifically the criteria I will use to evaluate the resumes of all candidates. What kind of successes do I wish candidates to demonstrate in a resume? Do I wish a candidate be a person of religious faith? Do I wish a candidate to have a strong position on the issue of abortion? Do I wish the candidate to have success in foreign relations? Do I want a candidate who has experience in operating a company or a government entity on a budget and has been successful in meeting the budget? Do I want a candidate who understands how to use key success metrics to identify the important things to measure and hold the government accountable for achieving?

I encourage each voter to do the same thing. I know what I don't want in a candidate: I don't want a media personality—a talking head that is photogenic. I don't want someone who only tests the way the political winds are blowing and who is governed by what political polls indicate will please the majority. I want someone capable of realizing they are applying for the most thankless job in the world—but the most important. Let's take the time to improve our role as voters and hopefully as organized political parties so we can bring to the forefront the most qualified applicants who clearly represent our view of "Presidential Material."

27

"An Alternative to Collective Bargaining"

Jonah Goldberg's **Register-Guard** article on **Union Busting in Wisconsin** (Thursday, February 24, 2011) made an argument explaining what he believes is a distinct difference between private-sector union battles with non-government business owners over employee "fair share" of profits, and public employee unions negotiating with agencies responsible for overseeing the public service funded by tax monies.

I am mulling over whether I buy his distinction. Of course his argument is colored by his belief President John F. Kennedy was politically motivated to strengthen the campaign funds Democrat candidates through such a decision. I am sure in the weeks ahead much will be written supporting and opposing Goldberg's perspective.

I hesitate to weigh in on this topic because of the mixed feelings I have about unions and unionization. My health care administration career began in 1974, the year the National Labor Relations Board (NLRB) ruled in favor of allowing health care employees to unionize. I never felt unions were "good" or "bad." I was taught unions played a positive role in shaping the American work-force. I was also taught unions were either "necessary" or "not necessary"—depending on the condition of the work-place and the quality of the organization's management and its relationship with employees.

I was vulnerable to the mythology that if employees unionized it was a sign of poor management. Such an argument did little except polarize anxious administrators into getting behind anti-union campaigns when a union collected sufficient interest cards to warrant an NLRB election.

For over two decades, I saw what amount to hundreds of millions of dollars spent on consultants who instructed hospital management teams across the health care industry how to wage effective anti-union campaigns when unions like the now well-established Service Employees International Union (SEIU) focused on the huge un-represented population of health care employees.

Perhaps it was fitting that as my career approached its end, the new President of my not-for-profit health care system (Catholic Healthcare West—a 40 hospital system based in San Francisco) decided to initiate a policy of not waging anti-union campaigns when SEIU or any nursing union raised sufficient interest among one of its hospital's staff to warrant an election. It was a radical change from traditional policy. Many old guard administrators felt the company had simply paved the way for the inevitable time when unions would take advantage of hospitals and financially run them into the ground. Such a prediction has not come to pass—though I am sure at least a few would say the jury is still out.

My administrative experience was only with collective bargaining in the **private sector**. On several occasions, my hospital organization went to the brink of strike-preparation with SEIU and the California Nurses Association (CNA) as we prepared to bring in temporary workers until the collective bargaining dispute could be resolved.

I have to admit that collective bargaining—however hostile and antagonist it became—eventually produced a compromise decision between union and management—sometimes through the help of a mediator or an arbitrator.   Collective bargaining serves a purpose, even though I look at the financial impact the strong SEIU and CNA presence has on the health care economy of California—as evidenced by the fact a full time benefitted dishwasher in my old hospital can earn in excess of $50 thousand dollars annually.   A non-specialized nurse approach and in some cases exceed the $100,000 mark.   Such wages and benefits must be put into the California cost of living perspective.

But the cost of labor is only one dimension of the health care finance problem.   I also grimace when I read the CEO of the not-for-profit system—a highly talented leader—earns in excess of $6 million dollars annually. Such a fact simply points to the incredibly complex financial, and some would say imbalance in the so-called not-for profit healthcare financial maze. But that reality must be resolved as a part of the other major national debate on health care policy.

In light of my private sector union experience, I now puzzle over whether collective bargaining with public employees is any different. I'm not sure whether Goldberg is overly simplistic when he asserts that *"government unions negotiate with friendly politicians over tax-payer money, putting public interests at odds with union interest. "*
If the Wisconsin political battle is about eliminating the right of public employees to collectively bargain, then

my question is this: "Is there really a viable alternative to collective bargaining for public employees? What is it? What did Jonah Goldberg mean when he said *"Government workers were making good salaries in 1962 when President Kennedy lifted . . . the federal ban on government unions? Civil service regulations and similar laws had guaranteed good working conditions for generations."*

I have long felt that in California (I can't speak for the pattern in Oregon) the tax-payers are to blame for the inflated cost of the PERS benefits. Instead of paying a market-competitive price for labor in the current economy, those who represent the tax-payers balanced annual budgets by withhold wage and salary increases with the promise of a richer contribution to a defined benefit retirement. Those who represented tax payers simply pushed forward the problem. The problem was not "collective bargaining"—it was how the tax-payers were represented in such a process. I do not fault any PERS retiree for becoming frustrated when someone threatens to take away something they have earned as entitlement. I am open to changing the deal for new folks, but not take-away from those who in good faith accepted a bargained contract.

So, to return to what I think is the question of the day, "Do we really have a viable alternative option to collective bargaining for public employees? " Should there be? If so, what is it?

28

"Snake Oil is still Peddled Right here In River City"

Caveat Emptor! Buyer Beware. Believe it or not snake-oil salesmen still traipse through Eugene. Even in economically strapped times—perhaps because of—con-artists continue to prey on folks looking for bargains that are—in fact—too good to be true.

We can never be reminded too often to be on the lookout and to expose such charlatans whenever possible. It is especially important when the spiel is slick and disarmingly simple to understand. I recently accompanied my wife to one such presentation. Hopefully, this will put others on alert to not check their critical thinking at the door when they accept invitations to such scams.

A post-card invitation set the stage. *"Come to the seminar. Listen to a 90 minute presentation. Even if you choose not to participate in our offer, just for listening to our sensational offer you will receive: 1) a coupon worth $300 dollars for gas; 2) two nights stay at a Marriot's hotel anywhere; and 3) two airline tickets to anywhere in the continental United States excluding Alaska and Hawaii."*

The travel company presentation was done at a reputable local hotel I will not name. It was a sunny day and the seminar was poorly attended—only one other couple. The articulate presenter joked that a couple of days earlier in Medford he had a standing room only response because it was raining. He said he was tempted to just give us the incentive reward packet and call it a day—at the least he could wrap up the presentation in 30 minutes—but he still used the 90 minutes on our audience of two couples.

What followed was a slide show that exploited common sense logic—his company didn't buy a dozen of rooms or a small block of airline tickets. They bought on a large scale—hundreds of thousands of rooms and tickets every year. *"Wouldn't you think you'd get a much better rate from such a high volume purchaser than shopping on the internet for your best price?"* The theme was reinforced with pictures of beautiful vacation spots and slides comparing supposed internet rates with what they could get—often 60% or more discounts.

Midway through the presentation the hook was set. In order to get these incredible deals, you needed to pay $5,999 dollars for membership in their club. Imagine if you had belonged to the club and what you would have saved in travel over the past three years! Imagine how much you could save in the future.

At the end of the presentation, each couple was assigned a supposed "non-commissioned salaried employee" to help us make our decision. I finally gave my firm "NO" and the salesman got the picture. He handed us the packet of incentives and erased the supercilious smile from his face.

Even the supposed "free" stuff was not without strings attached. When we got home I looked at the coupons. In order to activate the Marriot's coupon you had to send a check or money order to process your certificate. You also had to send money if you wanted to activate the airline ticket incentive coupon. Finally, if you wanted to get the $300 dollar gas value, you had to get approval for a service station in your home area and had to send in gas receipts totaling $100 each month— which would entitled you to a $25 dollar rebate coupon for additional gas. In other words, you had to spend $1200 dollars on gas over a one year period and submit receipts each month.

We tossed all the coupons. I went on the internet and found that the Florida –based company had received several complaints from disgruntled purchasers of the program.

In the final analysis, all the company was selling was membership in their service that promised to get good rates on future vacations. There were no price guarantees. In fact, there was no contract or agreement than any of the reduced bargain-rates displayed in the presentation could ever be obtained for you in the future.

The whole presentation was designed to create an illusion. You had to accept all the assertions and claims of spectacular savings and deals to be had at highly desirable vacation locations. You had to accept that they did in fact have the incredible volume discount purchasing power they claimed AND that the savings would be passed on to you without any mark-up.

I am not accusing the people who made the sales presentation of doing anything illegal. In fact, I am certain the company's attorneys have carefully trained the representatives to walk the fine line. Is such a scam unethical? All the presentation did was disarm a person's basic common sense approach by elevating the appeal to an emotional level. It preyed on people who want to get something for nothing—it preyed on folks who didn't ask the critical questions like, "What value do I really get for this $6,000 purchase?"

You wouldn't ever consider paying $6,000 dollars to join Triple A to access their discounts. Don't fall prey to such scams. If it promises something that is too good to be true or some incentive that is too good to pass up, buyer beware!

29

(**NOTE:** This is an opinion I sent Jack Wilson the week after Oregon played its heart out at the Rose Bowl. Given the scandalous events that followed in the months after the game, I am somewhat thankful that this essay never saw the light of day. I am since pleased to see that Mr. Masoli continued with his football career at Old Miss and was given a second chance. I'm just glad Jack Wilson probably knew something I didn't know about Mr. Masoli's lifestyle.

"Thank You Jeremiah Masoli"

Dear Mr. Masoli,

Thank you Jeremiah Masoli for your leadership that took the Ducks to the Rose Bowl and enabled local Oregon fans to enjoy what former University of Oregon Professor Edwin "Bing" Bingham called "healthy provincialism." Perhaps there is no better example of what Dr. Bingham described as one of the great virtues of our American culture—a local community's ability to celebrate and be boosters of a community spirit. We are blessed to live in a university town where such "healthy provincialism" thrives.

Like many Oregonians I made the effort to attend the Rose Bowl—a decision my old college buddy and I made over the phone fifteen minutes after you led the Ducks to victory in the Civil War game and clenched the Pac-10 title! Even though the game's outcome was not what I preferred, during the long drive back from my friend's home in Irvine, I had a chance to put the Rose Bowl adventure into a slightly different perspective than what was being processed by some disappointed sports fans.

For several hours I listened to radio programs where sports commentators opine about the game. I heard countless arm-chair quarterback analysis about what you could have done differently. I listened to "what if" scenarios about what could have changed the game outcome for Oregon.

Unlike some who viewed the game in terms of the statistics and the final numbers on the scoreboard, I had an entirely different take on the whole event. I was determined when I returned to Eugene I would write you and thank you and your teammates for giving your best in what I viewed as a great contest between two conference champions.

Mr. Masoli, I encourage you to return to your studies energized by the Rose Bowl adventure. I encourage you to look beyond the athletic competition and appreciate what you enabled through your athletic talents. One of the values of the Rose Bowl experience was how it fostered healthy provincialism in communities across Oregon. Healthy provincialism fosters human relationships and builds community identity and pride. It enabled humans to set aside temporarily concerns about all that divides the world along social, political, and economic differences. It celebrates our commonality and downplays at least temporarily our social differences.

I was among those who chose to travel via car down I-5 to attend the game instead of flying in and out of the sports venue. My choice allowed me to spend 14 hours of solitude driving back to Eugene from my friend's home in Irvine.

During the game I sat in the $145 dollar end-zone seats at the end of the field where the Oregon name was written on the turf. Much of the game, however, was spent on our feet, clapping and cheering on you and our team. I cheered and high-fived with complete strangers when the Ducks scored the touchdown that temporarily elevated hopes of victory.

When the game ended and Ohio State fans were jubilant with the victory, I felt badly for you and the Oregon team who had played so hard. I knew you and each player could not appreciate during the heat of competition was how much your efforts enabled and nourished each fan's network of relationships and enriched their individual Rose Bowl adventure and experience. In my case, I visited a family member home in Glendale I had never visited before. I connected with my ex-brother-in-law and half-brother (figure that out if you can) I had not seen in several years. I attended the game with another Oregon Duck who also received his graduate degree from Oregon. We again enjoyed the fellowship of attending a Rose Bowl game—and recalling our Rose Bowl experience from 15 years earlier!

I hope you and all of the Oregon players will now find time to reflect on the fact that your effort resulted in more than shaping the final score of an athletic contest. As you return to the classroom and your studies, I hope you will put things in perspective. I hope you can feel a sense of awe that 93,000 people sitting in the stands and enjoying your athletic efforts had their lives enriched beyond what the score reflected. You and your teammates provided a reason for so many to connect with networks of friends, neighbors, and family to create memories that will far outlast the memory of the final score of the athletic contest. I can't even imagine the millions of other relationships that were renewed and revitalized by those who gathered around television screens in homes across the country to share the common bond of being Duck fans!

I left Irvine early the morning after the game. Once over the grapevine and down into the flatlands of the central valleys of California, I was struck by how the Oregon license plates seemed to outnumber the California plates! Each time I stopped at one of the rest stops along I-5, I shared smiles and greetings from others who were clad in Oregon sweatshirts and who climbed back into cars and vans decorated with Oregon flags and colors. For 14 hours I saw an endless stream of cars and vans filled with Oregon families and friends making their way back to Oregon. Whether those Oregonians realized it or not, you and the Oregon football team gave them a winning experience far more valuable than the game's final score.

Thank you Jeremiah Masoli for enriching my life by enabling me to reconnect with family and friends and enjoy the contest you and the other Ducks waged in the Rose Bowl. I'm ready to do it again next year! Go Ducks!

30

"The Miracle on Pennsylvania Avenue"

I am surprised by two things: none of the political pundits who write nationally syndicated columns that appear in the **Register-Guard** have yet to assert President Obama is going to be successful in securing health care reform legislation—indeed, many remain skeptical. I am also surprised how none have dared to touch the obvious religious allegory in the drama unfolding in Washington these days—perhaps with good reasons: they don't want to raise the dander of the religious right that is already aligned with those who are hopping-mad about the pending health care reform legislation.

As a fiction writer/health care policy advocate, I have shared many strong opinions about the likelihood of successful reform. I am now willing to declare, however, that President Obama will be successful—for reasons that will soon be apparent. I also cannot resist point out the allegory between the events unfolding on Pennsylvania Avenue and the time frame that spans the Christian holidays of Christmas and Easter.

Recall it was on Christmas Eve, 2009 when the U.S. Senate stayed late into the evening to give birth to the Senate version of President Obama's health care reform bill. To say the Bill has suffered persecution and scorn from all sides is an understatement. That is why I can't resist the temptation to view President Obama Wednesday evening prime-time speech as his effort to resurrect and prove that there is life after death for the bill that many had abandoned.

Just as it was critical to get the vote before the Christmas break, it is likewise critical to the strategy of the Democrats to get a vote on the revised health care reform package before Congress is dismissed for the Easter break. Critics are upset. They charge such a tactic is clearly designed to buffer Congress folks who support reform from the hostility they will face from constituents who don't. History may well characterize the current health care reform drama as the "Christmas/Easter Miracle on Pennsylvania Avenue." True reform came to life—died several premature deaths at the hands of its crucifiers—then was resurrected into law during the week before Easter.

The political miracle, however, is only the precursor for what is to follow as Congressional reform-supporters confront the wrath of hostile voters who think the bill is too expensive, unaffordable, unfair to some segments of the health care industry and too generous to others. There is no question many legislators are putting themselves into political harm's way through their votes. I would like to think, however, that those who vote their beliefs and lose their jobs will have the satisfaction of knowing they didn't compromise their beliefs. Conversely, those who voted politically—and not in ways that reflect their beliefs—they will pay the greater price in losing their integrity and satisfying their self-interests. I sympathize with Congress members who challenge themselves with the adage, "If not now, then when?"

What about President Obama? Does the passage of the health care legislation signal his demise as a politician? As a politician, Obama desperately needs to win this debate. He needs Speaker Pelosi to cut the deals—forget about transparency. Make no mistake that this is about to happen.

Obama can still maneuver the votes—at least for now. All the ranting and raving of outraged Republicans cannot stop a health care bill from reaching the President's desk. The only thing the minority party can do at this point is to lick their wounds, cry "foul" and get folks focused on defeating the Democrat's majority in the upcoming mid-term elections. President Obama is well aware such a reality is apt to happen whether the reform bill passes or not. That's politics as usual.

The mid-term elections are—in the Grand Scheme of Things—the least the current administration has to worry about. That's why President Obama is willing to forge ahead with his agenda. He knows he is damned if he does and damned if he doesn't when it comes to health care legislation. So why not do what he thinks is the right thing for the country and move on with the rest of the agenda? What is there to lose?

The real test of the Obama administration's worthiness to move beyond a single-term presidency is not going to rest on the success of a health reform bill—however little or much is actually pared down in the President's final version. If the President doesn't score big on jobs, on addressing deficit, winding down the unpopular wars, and strengthening national security, then universal health care access for unemployed, insecure, war-plagued, and deeply indebted American's will not be viewed as a miracle but something that is exacerbating an economic nightmare and foreshadowing a grim future for America.

Covering 30 million more Americans with basic health care access is not going to change the ugly mood among the American voters towards our government's political process. The process, however, hasn't changed. What has changed is the awareness level of the American people toward how the process works. It isn't broken. It continues to work as it has always worked. At this moment in time, the Democrats dominate. They have the power to make the deals—and they will, rest assured! That's why President Obama will have a health care bill on his desk before the Easter break. That's always been the true miracle of Pennsylvania Avenue—that anything so big and consequential can actually get done.

31

"Re-Defining the Political Meaning of *Entitlement*"

The current debate regarding raising the national debt ceiling is going to require Democrats and Republicans to re-define the political meaning of *entitlement*. The Random House Webster's Collegiate Dictionary defines *entitlement* as the right to guaranteed benefits under a government program.

There was a time in American culture when we talked about "welfare" and in so doing the concept garnered a pejorative sense—a stigma was associated with welfare because people equated it with a government hand out.

The tradition of rugged individualism and self-sufficiency and being responsible for one's own well-being gave way to the realities that the modern economy was not a level playing field for all players. The movement away from the security of a farm and/or a family business in an agrarian culture into an industrialized urban settlement created unique problems for struggling Americans looking for ways to support and grow families.

When our parents and grandparents faced the economic realities of the Great Depression many people felt ashamed of being "on the dole" and having to swallow their pride and accept money from the government to make ends meet to raise their family. Few people saw such funding as being "entitlement" and even fewer wanted to remain on the dole any longer than necessary.

The term "entitlement" softened the reality that government programs had any stigma. With the expansion of government over the past several decades, countless "welfare" programs have permutated into "entitlement" programs—and as a society we have learned to accept this growing segment of our American socially-engineered economy as a necessary reality.

I am an American socialized into believing that "entitlement" is separate from "need."

I am also a retired person over sixty-five and "entitled" to both Medicare and Social Security benefits.

I confess I took early retirement Social Security benefits at age 62. Why? Because I feel "entitled" to the $1600 dollars a month I get from Social Security—and I was worried if I didn't sign up, I would lose this "entitlement" I had **earned**.

Now I introduced a new term, "**earned**." That concept makes "entitlement" much more acceptable for folks like me. If you **earn** an entitlement, it is quite compatible with the American cultural concept of individualism. Sadly, with the exception of Social Security and Medicare, there are few "entitlement" programs that one earns.

I earned (paid into the fund) my social security benefit and therefore I am entitled to it. Period.

Such thinking must be modified. It is time to ask me, do I "need" my social security benefit? If I do, then fine, let the entitlement program send me a check. If I don't meet a means test, then stop payment. That is a reality many of us middle-class and above recipients of social security must come to terms with if we wish to help America survive through these difficult economic times.

Stepping away from Social Security entitlement, I need to look at my Medicare "entitlement" as well.

I want to have health care insurance. When I was employed I paid a portion and my employer paid a portion of the cost of a comprehensive, standard insurance policy. When I retired, I transitioned to a government "entitlement" program Medicare and a supplemental insurance that allowed me to continue with the same type of coverage I enjoyed as a privately insured insurance enrollee.

I think we have approached the point in the American economic model where we also have to ask Medicare entitled patients to meet a means test to determine how much the individual must pay and how much must be borne by the government. Medicare must be based on needs and not on entitlement. This is going to be a major cultural transformation that will be hard for some Americans to accept.

I also am a great advocate of requiring anybody covered by Medicare benefits to participate actively in managing their own health status. If a person is unwilling to participate in pro-actively managing their health care risks and subsequent intervention care protocols, I advocate they should not be considered part of the solution because they choose to be part of the problem for the rest of us tax-payers who are footing the bill for some form of universal health care coverage.

These are extraordinary times that require each American to stop saying they are entitled to something when the reality of our current economic situation is such that we must all make new covenants if we wish the system to work for all of us in the future.

There are many of us who may well be "entitled" to Social Security and Medicare benefits—but we may need to make an additional sacrifice for the common good of our entire society. My only concern is that we find tools to means test that are equitable and spread the responsibility to make sacrifices across the entire spectrum of the American people. I don't want to make the sacrifice if others don't follow suit.

I don't want us to become a society like what we see in Greece. If everybody is entitled to virtually everything, then there is no challenge or opportunity for anyone to use their unique gifts as an individual and acquire wealth and prosperity that is the cornerstone of a capitalistic economy. Sadly, governments can build dependency on government by creating an "entitlement" mentality because it cultivates a dependency mentality.

Let us equate entitlement with "need" and get away from the concept that entitlement can be "earned." Let us stop making people dependent on government for things they should do for themselves. We can no longer afford entitlement programs in their current form.

32

"The Sad Reality of the Weiner Resignation"

I am not among those celebrating the resignation of disgraced Congressman Anthony Weiner. I was saddened to learn about his internet social media follies. One would think a 46-year-old recently married man with a pregnant wife would have more commonsense! Congressman Weiner represents the sad reality of politicians who confuse political power with sexual prowess. Maybe it is time to place heavier value on electing female politicians over male opponents—all else being equal in their qualifications?

Is philandering a **male** politician character flaw? Do female politicians scandalize their career and marriage relationship because of inappropriate sexual behavior? Are Democrats more prone to such behavior than Republicans?

In studying these questions at the Congressional level, I learned that the Constitution gives the Senate the power to expel any member by a two-thirds vote. In the list I studied more democrats were expelled than republicans. 23 democrats were expelled or censured; 10 republicans—the most recent being Oregon's Robert Packwood, a republican who was charged with sexual misconduct and abuse of power—he resigned before the Senate vote. Most of the earlier Congressional scandals related to loyalty, bribery, embezzlement, and corruption—and not sexual indiscretions.

Looking beyond the halls of Congress, I found a list of state and local political sex scandals in the United States. The list was revealing: Schwarzenegger, California (R), Hooper in Wisconsin(R), California Assemblyman Duvall (R), California Mayor of Los Angeles, Villaraigosa (D), California Assemblyman Samuelian (R),Florida State Representative Allen (R), Kansas Attorney General Morrison (D), Kentucky Governor Patton (D), Louisiana Senator Vitter (R), Louisiana State Senator Thomas (R), Nevada Governor Gibbons (R), New Jersey Governor McGreevey (D), New York Governor Spitzer (D), South Carolina Governor Sanford (R), and Tennessee State Senator Stanley (R).

This list is not exhaustive, but illustrates how no political party owns credit for having more philandering politicians—and, neither party seems better prepared to hold their members accountable for such indiscretions or to curtail the trend. It annoys me how the Wiener affair has provoked both political parties to focus on charging the other with being more tolerant of their own party's indiscretions than they are of the opposing party's indiscretions! Such argument speaks volumes about American politics!

After my investigation I am inclined to draw this conclusion: even though elected female politicians in high public offices is a relatively recent trend, they seem to be more focused on dealing with the policy issues they were hired to address than their male counterparts.

The tendency of females being less involved in sex scandals than male politicians can easily be explained by the numbers. Cynics may say, just elect more females and give them enough time and they will fall prey to the temptation of confusing political power with sexual prowess!

I'm not sure such a view is warranted, however. In my brief survey of sexual scandals among politicians, I only found reference to one female at the State level involved in a sex-related political scandal—Utah State Representative Katherine Bryson (R), in 2004. That doesn't mean others are not involved, but the trend appears quite obvious: men do it more than women. Why? I will leave such an answer to people more qualified than I am to suggest plausible hypotheses.

I write fiction so the philandering politician served as fodder for one of my plots.

A few years ago, I published a novel **THE IRON BUTTERFLY**. (Still available on Amazon.com) It told the fictional story of a tell-all book published by a dying woman in Washington DC. She was a well-known political campaign manager who was well aware of philandering politicians. She accidentally uncovered a governmental agency set up to protect congressmen against their own worst enemy—their inability to distinguish their political power from their sexual power. The story evolved around proving the existence of a clandestine government agency called "the second secret service." Its purpose? To provide a government sponsored escort service to politicians so they could discreetly engage in their inappropriate sexual behavior outside the limelight of the media.
I certainly don't advocate such an institution in the real world. Politicians like Weiner demonstrate, however, how the problem is ongoing. I hope Weiner is able to address the flaw in his character and find effective professional help. Sadly, I don't have any

recommendation for how either political party can effectively manage this problem among its members.

In the meantime, I am joining the ranks of folks who believe female politicians bring something to the public office missing in males. That doesn't mean I advocate electing a female over a male simply because of gender. However, unless we find some way to curb this inappropriate behavior from male political figures, the public may give the gender issue higher consideration than it has in the past.

I am reminded of something attributed to the former female governor of Texas, Ann Richards. She touted the choice of females candidates over males when she said, "If you give us a chance, we can perform. After all, Ginger Rogers did everything Fred Astaire did—she just did it backwards and in high heels."

The actions of people like Congressman Wiener, and governors Schwarzenegger, Spitzer, Sanford, and John Edwards certainly makes me pause and give serious consideration to voting for a female candidate when evaluating equally qualified male and female candidates.

I am tired of listening to resignations and apologies by disgraced politicians. Electing more qualified female candidates certainly mitigates this disgusting problem.

33

"Farewell Encyclopedia Britannica"

(**Note**:   I think this was an article that interested
Jackman Wilson but one of my submissions on health
care bumped this piece! And, after the announcement
of the closing of the publication was made, my lament
lost any of its timely appeal.)

* * * * * * * *

I was saddened to receive word from an old colleague about the recent passing of a venerable old
piece of American cultural history. Sometime in
the first couple of weeks of March, 2012, the printed
version of Encyclopedia Britannica was eclipsed by the
digital age of the internet and websites such as Wikipedia and a host of search engines that access information
instantaneously.
Many of us over-sixty-five folks have fond memories of
pulling down a heavy volume of the Encyclopedia Britannica and consulting its authoritative pages for
information we could included in our history, science,
or literature homework assignment. Some of us even
perused the volumes out of genuine curiosity to learn
something new about the world.
Many parents like mine who have since passed would
recall how they ushered into the front room of our modest post-war subdivision tract home a charming, well-
dressed door-to-door salesmen who convinced cash-

strapped young parents how shameful it would be for them to pass up the opportunity to use the simple monthly installment payment plan so their children could access the 32-volume set of attractively bound brown leather books with embossed gold lettering. It would assure parents their children would climb to the top of their class and excel in school for years to come.

I recall in my own history how I relied on the Britannica for information about George Washington that enabled me to win a $50 savings bond for an essay I wrote that won the first prize in the American Legion essay contest when I was in the sixth grade!

Somehow it seemed appropriate to include an obituary in tribute to this passing piece of Americana. I was among those who throughout my grade school and high-school years held the massive set of books in high esteem—although I recognize the world has changed and information storage and access was revolutionized by the internet search engines. Now students can be virtually anywhere and access information—not confined to the home study desk and the bookcase that held the volumes of the Britannica.

The printed edition of Encyclopedia Britannica enjoyed a long, robust life span of 244 years. The idea of such an educational resource came to life in 1768 when a Scottish engraver, Andrew Bell, and a printer, Colin Macfarguhar, created the first three cross-referenced volumes known as Encyclopaedia Britannian.

Unlike the often dubious entries of the modern Wikipedia, there was never any doubt about the authority of what was written in the Britannica. Over the years it had articles by Marie Curie, Albert Einstein, Henry Ford, and a host of other esteemed and respected authorities.

The popularity of the set of books reached a zenith in 1990 when the company sold 120,000 printed sets. In

2010 the company printed 12,000 sets and only sold about a quarter of that printing. The 32-volume set sells currently for about $1,500 dollars.

As a writer I continue to cherish the high touch experience of a printed bound version of any book. I am, however, not totally a printed book Luddite. I sell some of my books as e-books and assist other authors publish their own works through print-on-demand companies. The passing of the printed version of the Encyclopedia Britannica again underscores for me the change in how we store, consume and share information.

I realize, too, that for several years I have had a copy of the Encyclopedia Britannica stored on my laptop computer. It was a sales incentive used to convince me to purchase the brand of laptop I selected. Except for loading the software into the computer initially, I have yet to return to the data base. Instead, I have developed the habit of using an internet search engine to answer the questions I would have turned to the encyclopedia to answer fifty year ago when the Britannica ruled my world of knowledge.

In fairness to the Chicago-based publishing company of Britannica, it should be noted they have re-invented their business and now make the majority of their profits through the sale and distribution of instructional programs in math, science, and the humanities.

Any obituary should put the history of the Britannica into its proper context. It was born EIGHT years before America became an independent country! It lived a long and prosperous life—longer than most literary institutions.

It has indeed transformed in the sense that half-a million households still subscribe to internet full-access to the Encyclopedia Britannica—and more than 100 million people still have access to Britannica in schools, libraries, and colleges.

The passing of the printed version of the Encyclopedia Britannica is a bit of nostalgia for some of us who can still recall with delight thumbing through various volumes on a rainy day intrigued by bits and fragments of new knowledge—and making the vow we never kept that someday we would read the whole set from A-Z. That was before television had more than three channels, and long before interactive games infected the current generation of young students.

34

"Paying Colleage Athletes"

(**NOTE:** In recent years more attention has been paid to debating the issue of whether college athletes should receive more of the economic value they bring to their school's athletic coffers. I solicited this article among friends and it stimulated a lot of impassioned debate on both sides of the issue. There was not sufficient interest on the part of the Register-Guard to warrant its publication in the local paper. I suspect the reason was that I have no standing in opining on sports issues—unlike my standing in commenting on health care.)

* * * * * * *

College Football: A Modest Proposal

When Jonathan Swift wrote in 1729 his **Modest Proposal** he satirized a solution to poverty in Ireland by suggesting citizens consume unwanted children as a source of tasty protein! The following modest proposal to reform collegiate football will surely be considered absurd by purists. Some will see it as cannibalizing the darling child of

American amateur athletics—the so called "student-athlete."

The problem with the status quo is that everybody except the amateur athlete makes money on the business enterprise. We are already eating our young football athletes and not paying a market price for the flesh we are consuming!

It is time to address this inequity. It is time to cannibalize a flawed economic model that has evolved in NCAA Collegiate football. It is time to recognize we have transformed amateur collegiate football into a business enterprise that is driven by "athletes-who-must-be-students" and enrolled in a university instead of the original intent of having "student-athletes" exchange their athletic talents for a full-scholarship leading to an academic degree.

Most Division One football programs place high priority on graduating "student-athletes." The higher the number of graduates the bigger the recruitment boast the program can make. I propose that if we changed the status quo, then such a criterion becomes irrelevant. The success of a program would be measured by how many athletes matriculated to the next level and go on to an NFL team. The really interesting statistic would be the percent of players who actually chose to go to the university where they played on its sponsored club team! Imagine how novel it would be that occasionally a real "student-athlete" would emerge and be championed as an actual student at the sponsoring university!

I love to watch Oregon football. I don't advocate that the University of Oregon stop "sponsoring" a football team—just sponsor it under a different model. Don't require athletes to attend the university. Agree to reformulate the leagues and uncouple teams from the idea they are championing "student-athletes." Call it what it is—a feeder league for the NFL. Pay the market price for the athletes coming from the talent pool created by the nation's high school leagues.

How much would it cost the University of Oregon, for example, to recruit and retain a Lamichael James—or a Darrin Thomas—legitimate Heisman Trophy candidates? How much would Stanford have to pay to retain the services of Andrew Luck?

The status quo of NCAA football at Division One doesn't actually eat its young—it simply subject them to indentured servitude and prevents them from earning a piece of the true economic value they provide the business of Division One NCAA collegiate football.

The case was recently made in the **Register-Guard** that for many of the "student-athletes" on the University of Oregon football team there is indeed an economic quid pro quo—a $30k to 40k a year economic benefit of a full-ride scholarship in exchange for the time they put in on the gridiron and the off-season hours of conditioning and preparation.

In order to initiate a method to level the playing field for all NCAA Division One teams who wished to convert their current program into a new pro-college football league, it would be necessary to have the NCAA role transform into a league model analogous to the NFL. A draft of high school talent would have to be initiated. The athletic departments would prepare themselves for the draft and do as the professional teams currently do in the NFL draft. It would be the league's responsibility to find ways to assure parity and competitiveness among member teams.

There would no longer be the current rules of NCAA recruitment and selection process. Families who want compensation for their talented high school athletes would no longer have to be ashamed of asking for under-the-table, illegal signing bonuses! Universities would not have to play the game of selling families on the virtues of the university's educational program.

NCAA Division One football athletics is the "business/entertainment" subsidiary of the university. Such enterprises have a separate budget, a different pay-scale, and are considered a partner in the University by helping student-athletes achieve their educational goals. Football is not the "core business" of the university— nor should it be treated as such regardless of the pressures from some alumni. In order to separate the educational mission from the entertainment subsidiary of the university we need to sever the football program from any pretense it exists for the purpose of allowing gifted athletes to acquire a college degree in exchange for sharing their athletic talents on the college gridiron.

It is time to move forward and agree that we will finally consume the dysfunctional ideal of the "student-athlete" and enjoy creating a University of Oregon sponsored pro-team that all alumni and future alumni who are football fans can enjoy saying "that's the pro-team the University of Oregon" is proud to sponsor.

It is time for such a modest proposal to get serious consideration. It is time we stop consuming for free the flesh of our collegiate athletes and provide them a piece of the action they justly deserve.